exerci
KT-545-403

osteoporosis

exercise plans to improve your life

debbie lawrence and mary sheppard

C015228281

Other books in the *Exercise Your Way to Health* series:

Back Pain
Arthritis
Type 2 Diabetes
Depression
Stress

osteoporosis
exercise plans to improve your life

debbie lawrence and mary sheppard

A & C Black • London

Note

Whilst every effort has been made to ensure that the content of this book is as technically accurate and as sound as possible, neither the author nor the publishers can accept responsibility for any injury or loss sustained as a result of the use of this material.

Published in 2011 by A&C Black Publishers Ltd
36 Soho Square, London W1D 3QY
www.acblack.com

Copyright © 2011 Debbie Lawrence & Mary Sheppard 2011

ISBN 978 1 4081 3181 7

All rights reserved. No part of this publication may be reproduced in any form or by any means – graphic, electronic or mechanical, including photocopying, recording, taping or information storage and retrieval systems – without the prior permission in writing of the publishers.

Debbie Lawrence and Mary Sheppard have asserted their rights under the Copyright, Design and Patents Act, 1988, to be identified as the authors of this work.

A CIP catalogue record for this book is available from the British Library.

Acknowledgements

Cover photograph © Shutterstock
Inside exercise photographs © Tom Croft
Inside photographs © Shutterstock, except on page 56 © Getty Images
Illustrations by Tom Croft except on pages 2, 17, 19 and 20
© Shutterstock
Designed by James Watson
Commissioned by Charlotte Croft

This book is produced using paper that is made from wood grown in managed, sustainable forests. It is natural, renewable and recyclable. The logging and manufacturing processes conform to the environmental regulations of the country of origin.

Typeset in 8¼/12 Trade Gothic by Saxon Graphics Ltd, Derby

Printed and bound in China by RR Donnelley South China Printing Co

contents

acknowledgements

The publishers would like to thank the David Lloyd gym in Cardiff and Debbie Lawrence, Mary Sheppard, Jenny Burns, Rob Burns, Ben Burns, Mary Sparks and Paul Conway for their kind assistance with the photo-shoot.

Writing and teaching are my passions and I am thankful to Charlotte Croft of A&C Black for asking me to contribute to the *Exercise Your Way to Health* series. What I hope for this book is that it reaches the people who it can help and that they are able to glean some valuable information from what is written and from the exercise ideas, to improve the health of their bones (and health generally) by making positive changes to their lifestyle.

I give special thanks and appreciation to my partner, Joe, simply for being the person he is.

I also give thanks to my co-writer, Mary Sheppard, who truly is an inspiration for being active.

I give thanks and gratitude for the gift of my own health, especially as my body ages.

Debbie Lawrence

I've been lucky to be involved in fitness for nearly 40 years, teaching, tutoring and developing courses. Exercise and fitness have given me so much and I hope I can pass on some of my enthusiasm. Taking small steps to improve your own quality of life is a very positive and rewarding experience. It needs some determination and often friends or family to help you stick with it. I wish you well on this journey.

My thanks go to all my family, who constantly inspire and encourage me, and especially to my little grandson, Gryff, who is just taking his first steps in life.

Debbie Lawrence invited me to work with her and I have much to learn from her writing experience. I am grateful for the opportunity she has given me.

Mary Sheppard

foreword

The benefits of exercise for our mental and physical health have been well known since ancient times (the phrase 'A healthy mind in a healthy body' was coined by a Roman poet over 2000 years ago).

In spite of this knowledge, the Western world is plagued by high levels of illnesses that could have been prevented through a simple combination of good diet and exercise. I have been a GP in a large urban practice for 30 years, and have watched in dismay as our prescribing rates rise year after year in a futile attempt to accommodate this.

But prescription medicine is often not the answer – or at least, not the only answer. Many studies have shown exercise to be an extremely effective method of preventing diseases such as osteoporosis. It also helps slow down the development of the condition for those who already have it. And exercise enables people to achieve a fitter, healthier body in general, as well as building a confidence and awareness that can help prevent trips and falls.

I thoroughly endorse this book. It shows in a clear and practical manner how to exercise safely and effectively if you have, or are at risk of, osteoporosis. In addition there is information on dietary and lifestyle choices that can contribute to an improved level of health in both body and mind.

Dr P. J. Harney MB BCH MRCGP

introduction

You've probably picked up this book because you have been diagnosed with osteoporosis, or you know someone else who has. It is designed to give you a brief insight into the condition, but more importantly to give you advice on what you can do to stop things getting worse. In particular, it provides a series of exercises that can be practised in your own home.

Exercise is vital for two reasons: it can create strong bones in the first place so that osteoporosis is less likely to affect us; and it also helps to maintain and build bone strength in later life when we may already have osteoporosis. In this way it can slow down the progress of the disease.

When we exercise, our muscles pull and tug on the bones and this stimulates the bone-building cells. Weight-bearing exercise is best – that is, exercise where your legs and feet bear your body's weight – which includes simple everyday activities like walking and gardening. It's also important to work on mobility, strength and balance, as these will help you stay steady on your feet.

The book is divided into three sections: the first provides an introduction to osteoporosis; the second part offers advice on a healthy lifestyle; and the final section provides well-illustrated exercises designed specifically for strengthening your bones.

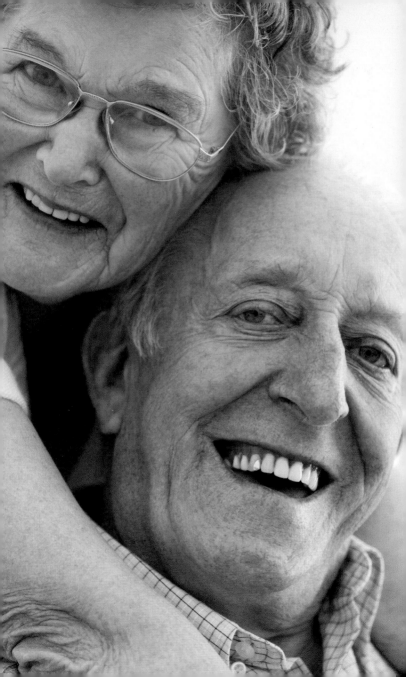

part

1

understanding osteoporosis

>> What is osteoporosis?

Osteoporosis, or 'brittle bone disease' as it is sometimes known, occurs when our bones lose some of the mineral content that keeps them strong and healthy. These changes make the bones more porous, brittle and susceptible to breakage. For those with osteoporosis, fractures and breaks can occur during normal activities that would not affect someone with healthy strong bones.

Health professionals differentiate between osteopenia and osteoporosis, depending on the loss of bone density apparent:

- **Osteopenia:** The early stage where there are mild changes in the thickness of the bones
- **Osteoporosis:** The more advanced stage

The chocolate-bar analogy

Imagine the structure of a healthy bone as being similar to a crunchy chocolate bar with the outside coated in a firm layer of chocolate and the inside like a honeycomb – strong but light, with lots of small holes and bubbles. For a bone with osteoporosis, the analogy is the inside of the chocolate bar after a mouse had been nibbling away at it. There would be lots of bigger holes, making the bar more fragile and more likely to break.

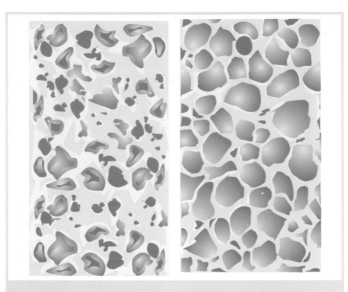

Cross section of a bone: (a) healthy (b) porous and brittle (osteoporotic)

> WHY DO WE NEED OUR BONES TO BE HEALTHY?

Our bones are essential for our daily functioning. First of all they provide us with our body shape – without this framework we would look like a jellyfish. Strong bones also help protect our vital organs:

- The skull protects our brain
- The ribs act as a cage to protect our heart and lungs
- The spinal column protects our spinal cord
- The pelvis protects our internal organs

Muscles attach to our bones, which act as a series of levers to help us move. During exercise, muscles pull and tug on bones and this stimulates bone-building cells, keeping the bones strong. The earlier you begin an exercise regime to strengthen your bones the better, but it's never too late to start.

Our blood flows through tiny blood vessels (capillaries) in the bones and delivers the essential nutrients like calcium that the bones need to grow strong. Exercise can help to improve the flow of blood to the bones, and the things we eat and drink determine the nutrients that we have available to nourish our bones. For example, milk and other dairy products are a great source of calcium and an important dietary requirement for people at risk of osteoporosis, as well as for younger people who are building healthy bones. We will discuss the beneficial effects of exercise and diet on our bone health in more depth in Parts 2 and 3.

BONE GROWTH AND DEVELOPMENT

Though we may tend to think of bones as being cold, hard and dry, they are actually constantly changing throughout our lives. Bones are made up of collagen (tough, elastic fibres) and minerals (gritty, hard material). However, they begin life as *cartilage*, which is a strong, rigid tissue that is softer than bone but hardens as the bones develop. Cartilage forms the shiny part at the end of bones, to protect the surfaces when they rub together. The end of the nose and ears are also cartilage tissue.

Our bones grow through a process called *ossification*. Calcium and other minerals are delivered to the bones to give us the right balance of spongy and solid bone tissue needed to form all the bones that shape our body.

- **Spongy bone** (cancellous) makes up most of the tissue within the bones that have a short, flat or irregular shape (e.g the collarbone, shoulder blades and wrist bones). It also forms the ends of the longer bones in our body (e.g. the bones of the arms and legs). Red and white blood cells are produced in the softer spongy bone tissue that contains bone marrow.

- **Solid bone** (compact) is the harder or more solid tissue that is deposited around the inner layer of spongy bone and gives the bones their harder and more compact property. Compact bone tissue provides support and protection, and helps the long bones of the arms and legs (the levers for movement) resist the weight-bearing stress placed upon them, in daily activities such as lifting, bending and walking.

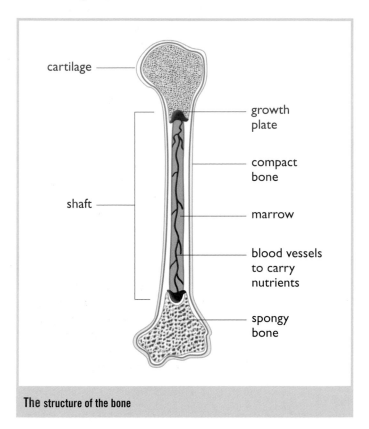

cartilage

growth plate

compact bone

shaft

marrow

blood vessels to carry nutrients

spongy bone

The structure of the bone

EMBRYONIC LIFE

Bones begin to develop while we are still in our mother's womb. A framework is formed from cartilage tissue, which gives the growing foetus its shape, and the framework developed during this time provides the foundation for our future bone development.

- **Osteoblasts** (bone-building cells) deposit layers of calcium along the length of the cartilage framework to produce a very thin layer of compact bone. The main shaft of the bone begins to take shape and form, but it is still soft so that a baby can pass easily through the birth canal.

- **Osteoclasts** (bone-destroying cells) remove any excess bone on the inner surface of the newly forming compact bone to prevent it from becoming too thick.

BIRTH

At around the time of birth, the growth plates (epiphyseal plates) between the main shaft and the ends of the longer bones are isolated. These plates remain as cartilage and become the main area for all future growth in bone length until we reach early adulthood, when they finally seal off and bone growth stops.

CHILDHOOD AND ADOLESCENCE

Babies often go through a period when they need to feed more frequently, and this is often linked to a growth spurt. Between the ages of 7 and 12 for girls and 10 and 14 for boys, youngsters often have a second period of fast growth. Bones grow first, giving longer limbs and bigger feet, often making young people appear gangly and uncoordinated. Fortunately, the muscles and the rest of the body eventually catch up.

Throughout childhood, the bone-building and bone-destroying cells work together in harmony to ensure that the correct balance of compact and spongy bone is developed. The activity of these cells is controlled by our growth and sex hormones (oestrogen and testosterone), produced by the glands (pituitary and thyroid).

EARLY ADULTHOOD

At the end of adolescence – around age 18 for women and 21 for men – our growth plates are sealed together. Our bones stop growing and so

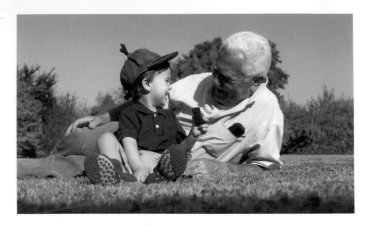

do we. By the age of 25 (approximately) our skeleton is fully formed and no further growth in length is possible. However, changes to the width and thickness (density) of our bones are still possible after this age. Without the right nutrition and sufficient weight-bearing exercise our bones will begin to lose density, but if we eat healthily and exercise regularly, our bones will stay strong.

> **WHY IS CALCIUM IMPORTANT FOR HEALTHY BONES?**
Calcium plays an essential role in the process of bone growth. It is also necessary for a number of other important body functions like blood clotting and hormone secretion.

The bones and teeth are our body's main depot for stored calcium but there are also small quantities circulating in the blood. The level of calcium in the blood needs to be maintained, because if it drops our body looks elsewhere for supplies of calcium – at which point it starts to break down the stores of calcium in our bones. This will happen regardless of how porous and brittle our bones are becoming.

Obviously it's important to keep the heart functioning, the blood clotting and the hormones regulated … but if this happens at the expense of our bones – because there is insufficient calcium in the blood – it will have consequences for our long-term health.

Calcium

In addition to its bone-building benefits, calcium plays a critical role in nerve transmission, heart function, blood-pressure regulation, blood clotting, hormone secretion and other body processes. This vital mineral can be found in readily available calcium-rich foods, including a few non-dairy options:

- Yoghurt
- Milk
- Cheese
- Sardines
- Salmon
- Cereal

- Tofu
- Almonds
- Rhubarb
- Spinach
- Brocoli and Kale

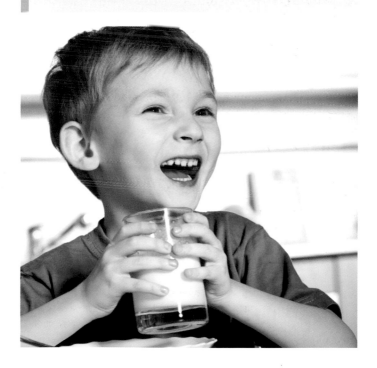

It's not a one-way process though. Once the levels of calcium in our blood have been restored – usually by absorbing minerals from foods like milk and cheese – another hormone called *calcitonin* stimulates our bones to reabsorb the calcium back from the blood. What this means is that getting plenty of calcium into your diet is an absolute must, both for creating and maintaining healthy bones.

Don't overdo it, though. The National Osteoporosis Society guidelines (2008) indicate that if you regularly have more than 2000–2500mg of calcium a day there could be medical implications. Too much calcium may also interfere with your intake of other essential minerals, like iron and magnesium.

Calcium content of some foods		
Food	Quantity	Calcium (mg)
Boiled spinach	4 ounces or 112g	179
Baked beans	4 ounces or 112g	59
Whole milk	1/3 pint or 190ml	224
Semi-skimmed milk	1/3 pint or 190ml	231
Ice cream	4 ounces or 28g	59

(Source: National Osteoporosis Society, 2008)

> > What puts me at risk of osteoporosis?

Osteoporosis is caused by a loss of bone density or *mineral mass*, particularly calcium. This happens naturally as we get older, but there are other genetic and lifestyle factors that will also affect our risk of developing osteoporosis. Here are some of the risk factors we cannot control:

AGE

Changes in the thickness and strength of bones are a natural part of the ageing process. The bones grow to a peak level of mass and strength up until the age of about 25–30. After this, both the mass and strength of the bones decrease.

The things we *cannot* change	The things we *can* change
Age	Inactive lifestyle
Gender	Smoking
Hormones	Diet
Body type	Alcohol intake
Ethnicity	Caffeine
Heredity	Fizzy drinks
Medical conditions / medication	Body-fat levels

The older we get, the faster our bones lose thickness and strength. The speed of this deterioration occurs at a rate of approximately 1% per year after the age of 30, and this rate increases further as we reach later life. It is estimated that by the time we are reach 50, one in two women and one in five men will have broken a bone as a consequence of osteoporosis (National Osteoporosis Society, 2006).

Starting early

It is important to be active and eat healthily when we are young because this will maximise the strength and mass of our bones. The stronger and thicker our bones grow when we are younger, the more we can potentially afford to lose in later life. However, the good news is that if we stay active, eat a healthy diet and have a healthy lifestyle (not too much smoking and drinking), we can actually slow down the rate at which our bones lose their strength as we get older.

GENDER

Women have smaller bones to begin with and are more susceptible to changes in the thickness and strength of their bones. Women also experience greater hormonal changes through their lifespan due to menstruation and menopause (see page 10). It is estimated that by the time women have reached the age of 70, they will have lost anything up to 30% of their bone mass (National Osteoporosis Society, 2006).

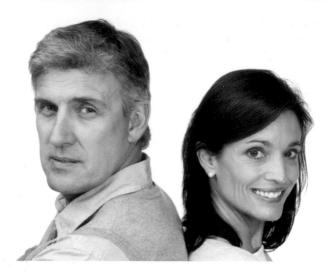

Most men have bigger bones, and they do not experience the same hormonal changes as women. This means there's a lower risk of them developing osteoporosis before the age of 70. For both men *and* women, however, other lifestyle factors such as being active, eating well and refraining from smoking, will delay or slow down the development of osteoporosis.

HORMONES

Hormone levels have a significant impact on bone health in both men and women. For women, the ovaries become active and produce more oestrogen when menstruation starts, and this helps protect the bones. During the menopause however, the ovaries stop working and stop producing oestrogen, which means that the bones lose their protection.

Women who experience an early menopause or undergo a hysterectomy before the age of 45 are more at risk of developing osteoporosis because of associated reductions of their oestrogen levels. On the other hand women who become pregnant benefit from an increase in the bone-strengthening hormone, oestrogen. Obviously women who don't become pregnant miss this particular opportunity to build up their bone density.

Although women tend to develop bone loss more quickly than men (approximately three times faster), men with low testosterone levels – known as *hypogonadism* – are also at a higher risk.

ETHNICITY

Caucasian and Asian women are more susceptible to developing osteoporosis, but it is less prevalent among women of African or Caribbean origin because their bones are bigger and stronger.

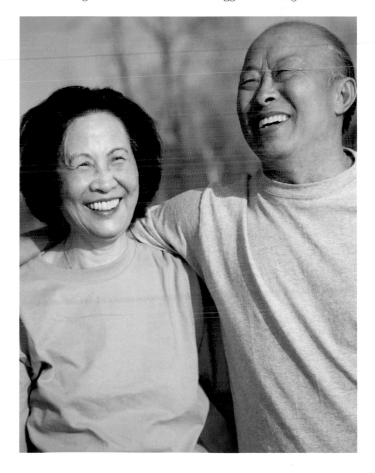

HEREDITY

If you have a maternal parent – in other words a mother or grandmother – who has experienced osteoporosis, then this will also place you at higher risk. Women who have a maternal parent with healthy bones and minimum breaks are less susceptible.

We also inherit our body shape from our parents. If our parents have a slender build and bones, we inherit this body type and an increased risk of osteoporosis (see below).

> My mother had osteoporosis and was dependent for most of her later life. I know there are hereditary links, so I am determined to keep my bones strong. I walk nearly every day for about 30–40 minutes and I train in the gym with weights on two days a week.
>
> **Rhiannon**

BODY TYPE AND BODY-FAT LEVELS

Women and men with slender body shapes are much more susceptible to osteoporosis than those with muscular or rounder body shapes. Those who have a low body weight for their height, and those with low body-fat levels, are also more at risk.

This is likely to be because slender body frames do not need so much muscle or body fat to cover the body frame. Reduced bulk and size and reduced muscle strength places them at greater risk of having lower bone density and developing osteoporosis.

Sometimes a woman's body-fat levels fall too low. This affects the production of oestrogen and therefore their menstrual cycle, which puts them at further risk. If in doubt, consult the height and weight chart opposite to see where you come on the scale.

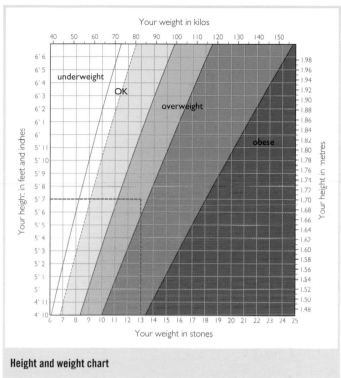

Height and weight chart

MEDICAL CONDITIONS AND MEDICATION

Our risk of osteoporosis is increased by:

- An accident or illness that causes a long period of immobility or bed rest, because we will not be active and building our bone strength during this time.

- Medical conditions such as Crohn's disease, coeliac disease and ulcerative colitis that affect the absorption of certain foods.

- Medical conditions that can affect the bones, such as overactive thyroid, rheumatoid arthritis, kidney failure and chronic liver disease.

- Eating disorders and conditions that affect the diet and interrupt the menstrual cycle and the production of oestrogen. Athletes who have to keep their body weight low are also at risk.

- Hysterectomies also affect the hormone levels that help keep our bones healthy and strong.

- Medical conditions that cause a reduction in testosterone levels in men, such as Klinefelter's disease or Kallman's syndrome.

- Gender reassignment, especially if hormone therapy is discontinued.

- Other medical conditions such as HIV (AIDS), organ transplants and respiratory diseases.

Medications that may increase our risk of osteoporosis include:

- Corticosteroids and anticonvulsants/epilepsy medication used to treat other medical conditions (corticosteroid tablets if taken for over three months)

- Treatments for breast cancer (aromatase inhibitors)

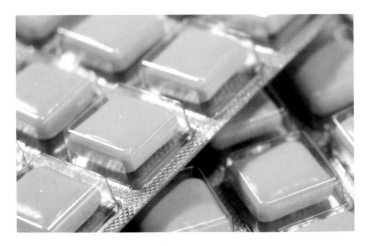

- Medication that affects the production or action of testosterone, such as treatments for prostate cancer

- Injectable progestogen contraceptives – medroxyprogesterone acetate (Depo Provera)

- Some medications used to treat mental-health problems (particularly medications for psychosis)

Many medical conditions are unavoidable. However, being active and maintaining a healthy lifestyle can help prevent some diseases like high blood pressure and coronary heart disease. This is another reason to start being more active as soon as you can!

> RISK FACTORS WE CAN CHANGE – THE GOOD NEWS

There are lots of things we can change to help improve the health and strength of our bones. These will be discussed in more detail in Part 2, but some key factors are described below.

> Inactivity (sitting down a lot and not moving our bodies) or a lack of weight-bearing exercise (walking or lifting things) will contribute to the rate at which the skeleton ages and our bones lose their strength and density. On the other hand, being active and taking exercise can help build strong bones and slow down the development of osteoporosis.

Inactivity causes the bones to become weaker and prevents the muscles from growing stronger. If you have ever broken a bone and had to keep it rested for 4–6 weeks, you will notice a big difference in the shape of the muscle when the plaster is removed. The muscles on that limb will already have begun to waste away. So you can imagine what years of being sedentary will do to both the muscles and the bones. Long-term inactivity and lack of use of the muscles will make us more susceptible to osteoporosis. Part 3 of this book will look at different types of exercise to keep your bones healthy and strong. Try to include some exercise in *your* life!

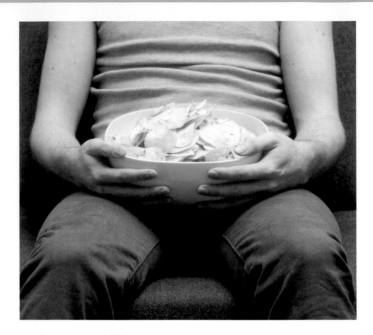

A balanced and nutritious diet is essential for keeping the bones healthy and strong and is another factor that we can change. A diet without enough calcium and vitamin D will increase the risk of developing osteoporosis: calcium is essential for bone growth and a number of other body functions, and vitamin D helps the absorption of calcium across the gut wall. Drinking too much caffeine, alcohol and fizzy drinks also increases the risk of osteoporosis, as these all prevent calcium being absorbed: choose healthier options such as water, juice and milk.

> ### WHAT KEEPS THE BONES HEALTHY?
Quite simply, to keep our bones healthy all we need to do is:

- Eat a healthy diet
- Keep our body active
- Take regular exercise
- Drink plenty of water
- Ensure there is calcium in the food we eat

- Cut out smoking and cut down on alcohol
- Limit our intake of coffee and fizzy drinks

If we are active, eat a healthy diet and reduce any negative habits we will be able to maximise the strength of our bones. If we are inactive and eat poorly, the health of our bones will suffer. Therefore it is essential to be active and eat well all through our lives, not just during the formative years. This is particularly important for post-menopausal women.

>> How do I know if I have osteoporosis?

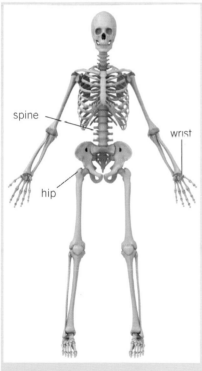

spine

wrist

hip

The three most common fracture sites

Osteoporosis develops steadily and progressively over several years without any noticeable signs or symptoms. It is some-times referred to as the 'silent disease' because it's hard to spot the moment where loss of bone density becomes critical. If you are over the age of 30, it is quite likely that you have some loss of bone tissue, but unlikely you will be aware of it.

The first sign is usually a bone fracture that you wouldn't expect to see if the bones are healthy. A knock that would only bruise someone with strong bones can lead to a fracture for someone whose bones have become porous through osteoporosis.

If this has happened to you, you should see your doctor as soon as you can. As well as helping you with a diagnosis and talking about the medical treatments available, he or she will discuss the amount of calcium and other essential nutrients that should be included in your diet.

Part of any strategy for managing osteoporosis should also include two other elements: minimising risks of future breaks and falls, and regular weight-bearing exercise. Both of these are covered in this book, so read on for support, ideas and tips on making positive changes to your health and wellbeing.

In advanced cases of osteoporosis, the spine can begin to crack and crumble and its shape can change. The upper-middle region (the *thoracic* spine) can be affected, resulting in a rounded upper back. This curvature of the upper middle spine, known as *kyphosis*, occurs due to an increased pressure being placed on the bones of the spine (the vertebrae). This causes tiny cracks and a wedge-shaped crushing.

A rounded upper back can restrict movement and mobility of the upper spine and may also cause breathing problems. In severe cases of osteoporosis, these factors may also contribute to fractures of the ribs and vertebrae in response to coughing.

One way to check your own risk of osteoporosis, prior to visiting a GP, has been developed by the World Health Organisation and you can find it on the National Osteoporosis Society website (www.nos.org.uk).

Their 'at risk' section will take you through a series of questions and calculate your risk of bone fractures and falls. This FRAX (fracture risk assessment) tool will lead you to the National Osteoporosis Guidance Group (NOGG), a source of further advice and information.

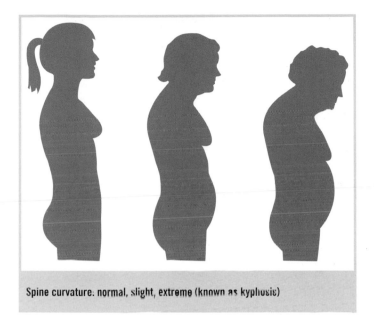

Spine curvature. normal, slight, extreme (known as kyphosis)

> ## HOW CAN OSTEOPOROSIS DIAGNOSED?

If you are concerned about your bone health, the best thing is to make an appointment with the doctor and try to get a diagnosis before any serious symptoms or fractures occur. The doctor can help you decide how to combat the progression of the disease through medication, diet and exercise, and advise you on your options.

There is no national screening programme in the UK at present. However, if you are a woman over 50, have gone through the menopause, and have several of the other risk factors mentioned in the table on page 9, your GP may refer you for a scan.

Called a dual energy X-ray absorptiometry – or DXA for short – this is a scan that can measure the calcium content of bones. Another newer test is digital X-ray radiogrammetry (DXR), which requires less technical equipment. It is not as sensitive as DXA, but may be used if you have perhaps broken a wrist after a fall. Using these scans, a health professional can determine whether you are in the early stages of osteoporosis (osteopenia) or the more advanced stage (osteoporosis).

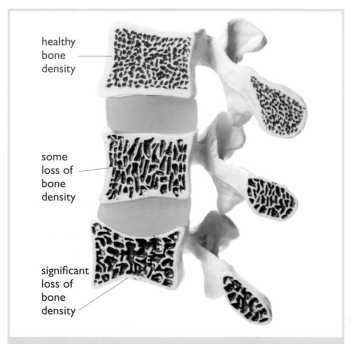

healthy
bone
density

some
loss of
bone
density

significant
loss of
bone
density

Spinal vertebrae showing normal bone density at the top, some loss of bone density (osteopenia) in the middle and severe loss of bone density (osteoporosis) at the bottom

> ## WHAT MEDICATION IS USED TO TREAT OSTEOPOROSIS?

Once osteoporosis has been diagnosed, there are a number of medications that can be used to treat it and your GP or medical professional will provide a prescription to suit your needs. The main types of medication currently available are as follows:

1. **Biphosphonates – alendronic acid or alendronate (Fosamax), cyclical etidronate (Didronel PMO), ibandronate (Bonviva), risedronate (Actonel) and zoledronic acid (Aclasta)**

These are the most commonly prescribed medications and are non-hormonal. They work by slowing down the cells that break down bone and enable the bone-building cells to work more effectively. Biphosphonates have been shown to reduce the risk of broken bones in the spine and, in some cases, the hip. They are used to treat:

- Post-menopausal women
- People taking corticosteroids for conditions such as asthma and arthritis

One side effect is irritation of the gullet, so they may not be suitable for people with stomach, bowel or kidney problems.

2. **Selective Oestrogen Receptor Modulators (SERMs) – raloxifene (Evista)**

These act in a similar way to oestrogen by helping to maintain bone density and reduce the risk of vertebral fractures. They may be prescribed to women only, to reduce the risk of spinal fractures and who cannot use biphosphonates.

> My grandmother and I get along like a house on fire. She's 72 years old, and I'm 21. Gran's been diagnosed with osteoporosis and has other health problems too. She takes regular medication, but also insists on the importance of being active – not just for her own sake, but for mine as well. 'Prevention is better than the cure,' she says! So every Saturday we go to the park and while she walks the dog I jog a few laps. And you know the best thing about it? Spending time with my amazing Gran.

Sara, aged 21

3. Strontium ranelate (Protelos)

This medication acts by impacting on the bone-building and breaking-down cells.

4. Parathyroid hormone (PTH) treatment (Preotact, Forsteo)

These work by building new bone and are only prescribed by specialists (not GPs) to people most severely affected by spinal fractures.

5. Hormone Replacement Therapy (HRT)

HRT using oestrogen replacement is prescribed for women during the menopause, as it can help maintain bone density and reduce fracture rates while it is being taken. It can also help reduce some of the side effects of menopause. However, HRT may not suitable for all women and is no longer the first line of treatment for osteoporosis. Prescription needs to be discussed with your GP.

6. Testosterone

This is the treatment to help maintain bone density for men with low testosterone levels (hypogonadism).

7. Calcium and Vitamin D supplements

Calcium and vitamin D supplements are most often used for those at high risk of osteoporosis and for whom bisphosphonates are unsuitable. These are especially beneficial to older people, as they can reduce the risk of broken bones and hip fracture. These supplements are also effective for people who are not very active and may not be getting enough calcium in their diet.

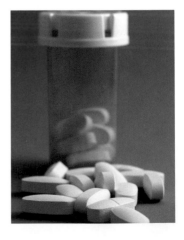

>> Preventing falls

As we get older we are all increasingly at risk of falls. There are a number of reasons why we may become unstable and more prone to fall:

- Poor eyesight and loss of hearing are very common and can affect stability
- Illness and some medications can leave people weak or dizzy
- Being less fit and strong overall affects our strength and balance
- Foot and leg pain caused by weakened ankles, sore joints, corns and so
- Urinary infections and bladder dysfunction

If you are concerned about falling, there are some safety suggestions on page 24. There is also information on getting up from the floor safely on page 64.

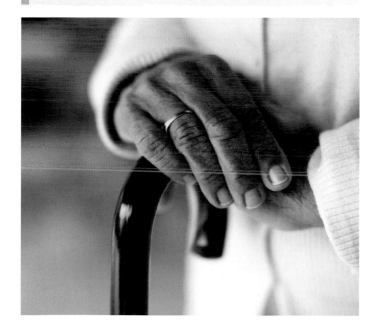

Common risks and how to reduce them	
Potential risk	**Strategy to reduce the risk**
Poor balance	Use a stick, walking pole or umbrella when on uneven surfaces. Do exercises to help improve your balance (see pages 83 and 103).
Poor eyesight and/or hearing	Have your eyes and hearing tested as both can contribute to poor balance.
Dizziness and light-headedness	These might be caused by low blood pressure – see your GP.
Medication	Some medicines, especially if taking more than four, may make you feel drowsy. If you feel more unsteady than usual, again talk this over with your GP.
Unsuitable footwear	Make sure your shoes support your feet and are suitable for you.
Worn or slippery surfaces and rugs	Check worn carpets and highly polished floors. Fix grippers to rugs to prevent slips and trips in your home.
Steep stairs	A second handrail might come in handy to give more support when climbing stairs. It is useful to keep using the stairs to maintain your leg strength.
Poor lighting and cold houses	Use light bulbs of 100 watts to give sufficient light and try to keep the house warm to prevent stiffness.
Clutter and trailing wires	Minimise clutter around the home and have any trailing wires safely fixed around skirting boards.
Icy and dark weather	Avoid going out when pavements are dangerous (during snow and ice) and take care on dark winter evenings.

Poor posture such as a hunched upper spine or kyphosis (see page18) also increases the risk of falling. The forward rounding of the spine creates a change in the centre of gravity that affects our balance, stability and co-ordination. In a case of this kind of advanced osteoporosis, take extra care and be vigilant. Use a walker and one or two sticks to increase your stability, and consider wearing a hip protector like the one pictured below, to protect you in the event that you do fall.

Even if you feel fit and strong you can still experience a fall, and the loss of bone strength that occurs as we age means that this is more likely to result in a break of fracture. Take a look at the table on page 24 to see how to reduce the likelihood of this happening. Prevention is always better than the cure, so it's well worth thinking about how to avoid common risks wherever possible.

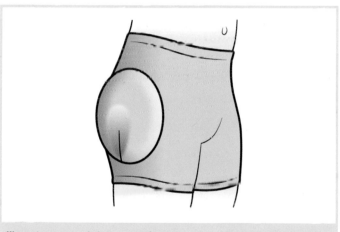

Hip protectors can help in more advanced cases of osteoporosis, cushioning your hips if you have a fall

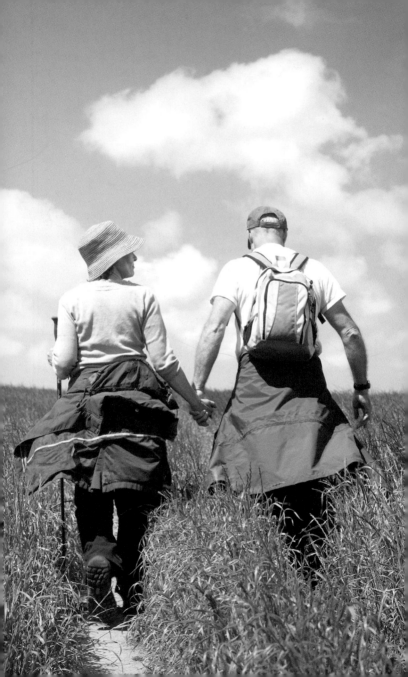

part

2

helping yourself to
health

>> The four-step strategy

Taking positive steps to help yourself to health will give you back some
personal power and help you to regain control, rather than letting the
condition control you. The greatest changes you can make to improve
your overall health and the health of your bones are simple and effective
lifestyle changes. Many ideas are given in this section of the book.

The four-step strategy that follows will help you assess your life, set your
goals, move towards them and stay motivated.

> STEP 1: WHERE AM I NOW?

The MOT questionnaire on page 29 is a simple checklist. It is not
designed to replace a medical check-up or advice offered by your
doctor, but it can help you identify the factors that affect you specifically,
and that might put you at risk of osteoporosis. And don't forget the
FRAX tool, endorsed by the National Osteoporosis Society and available
on their website (see box on page 18).

Go through the questionnaire, putting ticks in the 'yes' or 'no' boxes that
apply to you. The more 'yes' responses you give, the more risk factors
apply to you. Don't worry even if you have a great deal of 'yes' boxes

ticked – there are still ways to improve the quality of your life and combat the development of osteoporosis. However, it is advisable for you to visit your GP to discuss the situation and request a bone scan.

Once you have completed the questionnaire, turn to the key on page 30. This will help you work out which group you are in – low, moderate or high risk. We have used a traffic-light system to represent each group:

⬤ **Red** for those with advanced osteoporosis

⬤ **Amber** for people who have been diagnosed with osteoporosis

⬤ **Green** for those without any symptoms but who may be at risk

It is important to take the time to complete the questionnaire and work out your level of risk. It should help you with the management of the condition, and with setting suitable exercise goals for the group you are in. The traffic-light system will also guide you towards the exercises that are right for you, and safe too, when you come to Part 3.

Hips and health

There are approximately 60,000 osteoporotic hip fractures in the UK each year, and many people experience the debilitating effects and the loss of independence this causes. It means it is essential that we take steps to keep our bones as healthy as possible. And it's never too late to start!

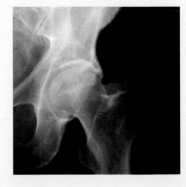

MOT questionnaire		no	yes
Answer the questions honestly and count how many yes and no responses you have			
1	Are you female?		
2	Are you over 50?		
3	Are you underweight?		
4	Do you have a slim body frame?		
5	Are you of Asian or Caucasian origin?		
6	Do you have a maternal parent with osteoporosis?		
7	Have you ever had prolonged spells without your menstrual cycle?		
8	Did you have a late puberty? (late starting menstrual cycle)		
9	Have you started the menopause?		
10	Do you smoke?		
11	Do you drink more than the recommended units of alcohol (see page 45)?		
12	Are you physically inactive, e.g not active on 5 days a week?		
13	Do you drink more than 6 cups of coffee a day?		
14	Do you drink lots of carbonated drinks?		
15	Do you have a sedentary job where you sit down a lot?		
16	Do you eat lots of fast food or ready meals?		
17	Do you have kyphotic posture?		
18	Have you ever broken a bone carrying out a simple daily activity?		

Level of risk

MOT	Diagnosis	Treatment plan	Exercise aim
Some *yes* responses	Low risk Healthy or normal bone mass or mild changes (osteopenia)	Start making lifestyle changes and being more active	• Focus on keeping the bones as healthy as you can to delay future bone loss • Most exercise programmes will be suitable unless other health conditions are present
Over 50% *yes* responses	Moderate risk You may have had a clinical diagnosis but without any history of fractures	Start making lifestyle changes Check with your GP before starting an exercise and activity routine. It may be that you need a medical intervention as well as making lifestyle changes	• Be more careful about the exercises you do, because of your potentially increased risk • You also need to be aware of the potential risk of fractures and falls
Mostly *yes* responses	High risk You may have had a clinical diagnosis and have a history of fractures	Start making lifestyle changes Check with your GP before starting an exercise and activity routine. It is likely that you will need or are already receiving medication to treat osteoporosis It may be that only **supervised exercise** is appropriate for you, via GP referral exercise schemes	• Be careful with all exercises and check with your GP first! • Aim to reduce your risk of falls • Improve your posture • Practise breathing • Some of the seated exercise suggestions may be appropriate for you, but do check with your GP first

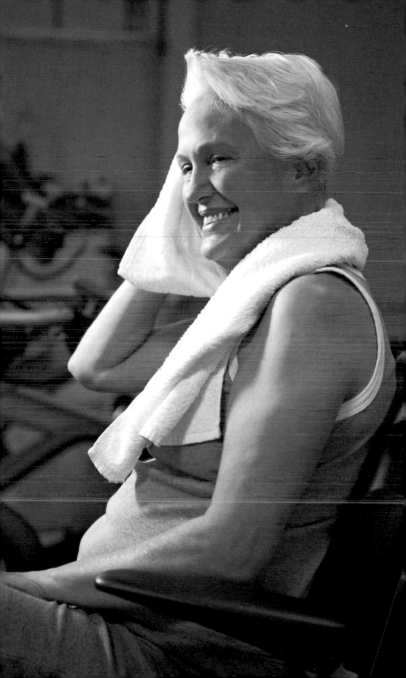

STEP 2: WHAT WOULD I LIKE TO CHANGE?

Look back at your answers to the MOT questionnaire. Have you ticked 'yes' for any areas of your life that you can change?

- Do you smoke?
- Are you physically inactive?
- Do you have a sedentary job?
- Do you eat processed foods and ready meals?
- Do you drink lots of coffee, carbonated drinks and alcohol?
- Are you underweight or overweight?

These are areas of your life that you can change. Choose one and make it your goal. It might be a challenging goal like stopping smoking, or something slightly easier like cutting down from six to four cups of coffee a day.

Before you decide, read through the rest of this section, including the lifestyle focus that begins on page 42. There is plenty of information and advice about how to improve different aspects of your life so that you are healthier, stronger and more able to combat the development of osteoporosis. Our aim in this book is to help you find a way that works best for you.

Try not to be too ambitious however, or you will make success harder to achieve. If you decide to stop smoking and start exercising at the same time, you are more likely to lapse. And slipping up can be demoralising, putting you off making positive changes in the future. It's best to take one small step and succeed at it. You'll find that each success spurs you on and gives you greater confidence in your ability to make changes.

Tips for setting goals

Write the goal down

Decide on a start date

Make it achievable

Take one step at a time

Reward yourself

If you do slip up, don't consider it a failure – forgive yourself and move on. Everyone does it – it's part of being human. Although it may be that you were being too ambitious to begin with and need to revisit your goals. Use the box below to help you:

Set yourself SMART goals

Specific: make sure you know exactly what you want to achieve

Measurable: think about how you will judge your progress

Achievable: have you given yourself enough time and support?

Realistic: make sure your goal isn't set too high

Time-framed: allow yourself enough time to achieve your goal
– it takes around 21 days to change a habit

> ### STEP 3: MAKING CHANGES
Now is the time to put your goal into action. Remember it is better to aim low and succeed than try to change everything at once and fail. This can involve taking a large and important goal and breaking it down into smaller parts:

- So rather than saying 'I want to get more active,' tell yourself: 'I would like to exercise for ten minutes after breakfast.'

- Rather than saying 'I want to eat a healthy diet,' begin with: 'I will eat an additional piece of fruit every day this week.'

Making changes seems far less daunting this way. And instead of putting them off, you might feel confident enough to start straight away.

Note: If your goal is to start being more physically active or to begin exercising, please remind yourself first about your level of risk – were you green, amber or red on page 30? We also advise you to go through the health questions on page 38. These are designed to highlight any other conditions that might affect what you can do – we would ask these questions of anyone who planned to become more active.

Are you ready to go? Have you set yourself a start date? Have you planned your approach? That's great! Don't expect it to be an entirely smooth road though. There will be bumps along the way…

> **STEP 4: HOW DO I STAY MOTIVATED?**

It can be hard to keep a commitment – even one you make to yourself. It's important to accept that there will be times when you relapse. When this happens, check that your goals are SMART (see page 33), then pick yourself up and try again.

Here are a few tips for helping you stay motivated:

1. **Be Smart.** Are you finding it really hard to stick to your plan? Perhaps your goals are not realistic. Go back to page 33 and check you've set yourself SMART targets.

2. **Get a friend involved.** It's a well-known fact that having *accountability* to someone – a friend who is expecting to go to an exercise class with you, for instance – is a very motivating factor.

3. **Know yourself.** If you find it hard to go out on a cold winter's day for a walk, set a target to do some simple chair-based exercises at home instead. If you can't cut down on the cups of tea you drink, take up drinking more water. Work with your strengths rather than trying to fight your weaknesses.

4. **Focus on the achievements.** Don't get obsessed with the things you have failed to do! People tend to do this, so it's important to look back and remember the many positive steps you have already taken – like buying this book in the first place.

5. **Reward the changes you make.** For short-term motivation, you could place a chart on the fridge, adding gold stars for the targets you achieve! For longer-term motivation, you may want to give yourself a bigger reward, like a holiday or a new coat.

6. **Write it down.** For example, if you want to start eating more healthily, you could use a food diary, or if you want to be more active, keep a weekly activity log (see the example on page 110). Plan what you want to do, and then record what you actually do. Keeping a daily log of your progress is very useful in many areas, and will help you when you come to reflect on your progress.

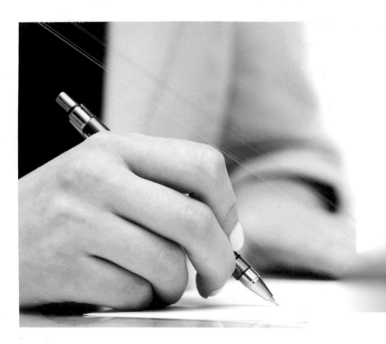

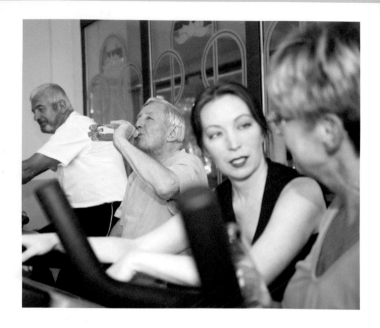

>> Exercise and you

There are so many goals we can set to improve our lives, from getting on top of the housework to finishing the book we got for Christmas. But most of us know that exercise really is one of the most important improvements we can make.

Some us take part in regular exercise, some of us start and stop, and some of us don't bother at all. Some of us have no time, some no inclination, and some don't feel physically able to exercise. If you want to make improvements to your health however, it is worth making the time for exercise. If you are worried because you are frail or unfit, you can always start gently with one or two exercises once a week. You can exercise from the comfort of your chair (see page 71).

Exercise·

- Increases the strength of the heart
- Improves the circulation of blood and oxygen
- Improves the rate at which we breathe
- Improves the tone and strength of our muscles
- Improves the strength of our bones
- Lowers blood cholesterol levels
- Lowers blood pressure
- Improves our mood
- Provides an outlet for tension and stress
- Reduces the risk of depression
- Burns calories and keeps us trim
- Improves balance and coordination

> My mother was nearly crippled with osteoporosis. The fractures in her spine meant she ended up bent right over and I was terrified I would end up like her.
>
> Then I found out that, through a few simple changes to my diet and taking more exercise, I could minimise my chances of getting osteoporosis, I started going to exercise classes in my early 40s and now I am in my late 60s and have no symptoms at all and feel fitter than I've ever done.
>
> **Chris, aged 67**

> ### ARE YOU FIT TO GET PHYSICAL?

Before you start taking exercise or being much more active, let's run through a few basic health questions. These are designed to highlight any other health concerns you may have, and it is customary to ask them of anyone who is considering taking up exercise.

Physical activity readiness questionnaire		yes	no
1	Has your doctor ever said you have a heart or vascular condition and/or that you should only do activity recommended or supervised by a doctor?		
2	Do you feel any pain in your chest when you do physical activity?		
3	In the past month have you had chest pain when you were not doing physical activity?		
4	Do you lose your balance because of dizziness or other reasons or do you ever lose consciousness?		
5	Do you have a bone or joint problem that is affected by or could be made worse by physical activity?		
6	Is your doctor currently prescribing medication for any condition?		
7	Are you over 69 years of age and not used to physical activity?		
8	Do you know of any reason why you should not take part in physical activity (sprains, breakages, recent falls, pain, etc.)?		

If you have answered yes to any of the questions please discuss the answers with your doctor who will advise you on whether it is the right time to become more active.

If you have answered *yes* to even one of these questions we would advise you to visit your doctor before you start taking exercise. This is just a precaution to make sure you do not aggravate an existing condition, or put yourself at risk when following a new fitness regime.

Don't worry or be downhearted about this – the key to making positive and safe changes is to start from a position where you have all the facts to hand. Exercise and activity can be tailored to any level of health and fitness, so there will always be something you can do.

Even if you have answered *no* to all the questions, there may be circumstances that mean that you should delay activity. These are:

- If you are unwell because of a temporary illness such as flu or a cold, wait until you feel better before becoming more active.
- If you are pregnant now or you have been pregnant in the last six months, you need to see your primary healthcare provider to check it is suitable for you to become more active.
- If you have been diagnosed with a medical condition in the last two months or are significantly overweight, you need to discuss becoming more active with your GP.
- If you are in pain or recovering from a fracture.

> > Being more active

The simple truth is that taking exercise is good for you in so many ways, including slowing down the development of osteoporosis. It's good for your mood, your waistline, your bones and your overall health. And it is never too late to reap the benefits, so there are no excuses for late starters.

However if the thought of joining an exercise class or even exercising in the privacy of your home is daunting, don't worry. You can always start by increasing your activity levels as you go about your day-to-day life.

But what do we mean by 'activity'? The answer is just about anything, from mowing the lawn to cleaning the windows, walking the dog to climbing the stairs. You don't need to grab a tennis racket or put on a tracksuit – you can simply get off the bus a stop earlier, or take a walk after lunch. Activity in itself is good for you: it's weight bearing and raises your heart rate, and this is a great place to start.

Ideas for getting active

- Walk the dog
- Walk with a friend
- Stroll down the road
- Visit the shops
- Climb the stairs
- Clean the car
- Put on music and dance
- Hoover the carpet
- Weed the garden
- Mow the lawn
- Park the car further away from your destination
- Join a walking group
- Get off the bus a stop early
- Walk up escalators
- Get out of your chair every half hour and move around
- Do chair-based exercises once a day
- Walk in your lunch break

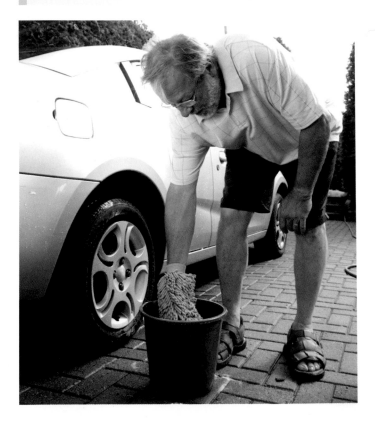

HOW MUCH SHOULD I DO?

It's a good idea to start being more active with a small amount on a few days – for example, ten minutes, three times a week. When you can comfortably manage this, increase the time and keep that going for a few weeks. Once that becomes easier to manage, start increasing the number of days on which you are active. You should be aiming for a programme like the one described in the table below.

Never forget: the key is to listen to your body. Remember, if you are not used to exercising and being active, start gently.

What to aim for when you exercise	
Frequency	Aim to be active on at least 5 days of the week. You can start once a week at first and steadily build this up.
Intensity	When you are moving, you need to work at a level where you feel a little breathless but comfortable. This will be different for each person: some people may find walking up the stairs easy and some may find it hard work. The goal is to select an activity that you can do comfortably and that makes you feel a little breathless.
Time	You should aim to be active for 30 minutes each day, but you can break this down into shorter intervals throughout the day while you are getting used to being more active. • Try starting with a short 10-minute interval of activity and repeating this 3 times during the day. It could be walking the kids to school or a walk to the shops or even around your own home. • You can then build up to 15-minute intervals of activity, twice during the day.
Type	Any activity that fits well into your daily lifestyle, that you like doing and that you know you have the potential to keep up!

Go outside!

An extra advantage of spending time outdoors being active is that 15 minutes of sunshine every day can really boost your vitamin D levels. These are important because they help you absorb calcium – essential for healthy bones.

> > Lifestyle focus

This section contains information on various ways you can make your lifestyle healthier. All of them can play a part in combating the effects of osteoporosis, either directly or indirectly – so for example, getting plenty of calcium in your diet is an essential weapon for slowing down the development of the disease, while sleeping well at night can keep you alert and help prevent falls.

> HEALTHY EATING

There are no bad foods per se, just poor diets. Too much of any food would be bad for you because you would not get all the nutrients needed. Take for example the 'grapefruit diet', used for weight-loss

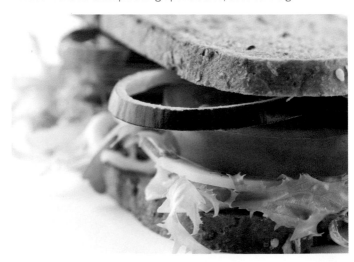

purposes – the fruit is healthy in small amounts, but it would not be balanced if it made up most of your diet. You would feel weak and lethargic, and after a while your health would suffer.

Take a look at the plate of food in the illustration below. This reflects the ideal balance of the foods in your diet:

- Fresh fruit and vegetables, and plenty of *carbohydrates* like bread, rice, pasta and potatoes, should make up the bulk of your diet.
- Proteins like meat and fish along with dairy products should make up a smaller proportion.
- Sweet things like cakes and biscuits should make up only a tiny segment!

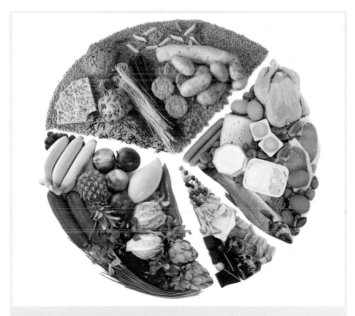

Balancing the food groups

Osteoporosis and food

The body contains 1kg of calcium, 99% of which is stored in our bones and teeth. There's also a very small amount in your blood that is vital for all sorts of functions.

It really is important to eat plenty of foods rich in calcium to help build or maintain healthy bones, and to stop your body breaking down your bones to get at the calcium stored there (see page 6). Vitamin D is also vital, as this helps with the absorption of calcium and other nutrients.

In fact, the Food Standards Agency recommends eating five different portions of fresh fruit and veg a day. This can be quite hard for people to fit into their diet, especially if they are busy. Try to keep fruit to hand for healthy snacking and eat a salad and fresh vegetables as often as you can. Even a glass of fresh fruit juice can count as one of your five-a-day.

Try to boost your levels of calcium and vitamin D by including some of the foods listed in table opposite in your daily diet. For example, you could increase your intake substantially by switching from toast to porridge or cereal for breakfast. You could even use milk fortified with calcium and vitamin D. Note that the calcium content of cheese varies a lot – Gruyère cheese, for example, has 50% more calcium than some hard cheeses, while cottage cheese contains more than cream cheese. For those who are lactose intolerant, there are non-dairy options too.

> I knew I was at risk of developing osteoporosis as I had chronic kidney failure in my early thirties. After the transplant I visited my GP to discuss it. She told me there were simple ways to build up my bones and slow the development of the disease. Now I monitor my calcium intake, and I exercise regularly. Like anyone else I may not escape altogether, but I know I've done my bit to protect myself and that makes me a lot happier.

Guy, aged 39

Foods rich in calcium and vitamin D	
Calcium	**Vitamin D**
Yoghurt	Salmon
Milk (calcium fortified)	Mackerel
Cheese	Sardines
Sardines/salmon (canned with bones)	Pilchards
Cooked rhubarb	Herring
Spinach	Trout
Tofu	Tuna
Almonds	Liver
Beans (baked or boiled)	Egg yolks
Broccoli/kale	Fortified milk or orange juice
Wholewheat bread	Fortified margarine
Breakfast cereal	Spinach
Dried fruits, e.g. apricots and figs	Watercress
Soya	Sesame seeds
Oats	Soya
	Almonds
	Tofu

There are many other vitamins, minerals and nutrients that are important for your health, and there is plenty of information out there if you are interested in finding out more. As a general rule of thumb though, if you eat a wide variety of foods, you will generally get a balanced mix of all the vitamins and minerals you need.

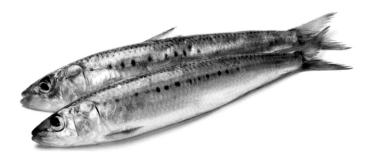

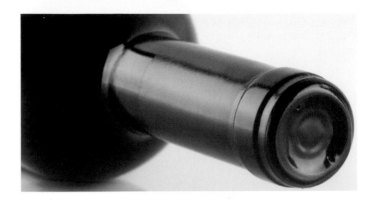

> **DRINK ALCOHOL SENSIBLY**

Alcohol from time to time can be a pleasure and a reward. There is no reason not to drink in moderation – so long as you are aware of what is moderate and what is not. The table below shows the current daily limits as recommended by the Food Standards Agency. The table opposite tells you how many units there are in some popular drinks.

Maximum recommended units of alcohol		
Health risk	**Units of alcohol**	
	Women	*Men*
☺ No significant risk	2–3 units per day (no more than 14 per week)	3–4 units per day (no more than 21 units per week)
☹ Increasing risk	3 or more units per day on a regular basis	4 or more units per day on a regular basis

As you no doubt know, the long-term effects of alcohol misuse are detrimental to our overall health. As well as causing social problems, drinking too much increases the risk of liver damage and even some cancers. What you may not know is that excess alcohol also reduces the amount of calcium we can absorb in the bones. People with osteoporosis should be particularly careful, and of course everyone should be aware that mixing alcohol and medication is not advised.

There is a wealth of support out there if you are concerned about your drinking. See the end of the book for more information.

Units of alcohol in popular drinks			
Measure/drink		**Alcohol by volume**	**Units**
Half pint of ordinary beer, lager or cider		4%	1.1
Bottle of strong beer (330ml)		5%	1.7
Small glass of wine (125 ml)		12–14%	1.5–1.75
Large glass of wine (175 ml)		12–14%	2.1–2.45
Single measure of spirits		40%	1

THE EVIL WEED – REASONS TO STOP SMOKING

Smoking also prevents the absorption of calcium into the bones. This in turn reduces their mass and strength and makes them more prone to becoming brittle and porous, which leads to osteoporosis. And of course smoking increases the risk of heart disease and cancer too, as well as a host of other health complications.

The negative consequences of cigarette smoking on health are well known – you don't need this book to tell you it's bad for you. And yet many continue to smoke. Smoking is highly addictive and once started is not easy to quit. Some people stop without help and go 'cold turkey', but many others will need support to stop.

Fortunately, there are a number of support services available that can help those who want to quit smoking, including the NHS. A visit to your GP is a good starting point. Even if you find it really hard to quit, don't give up trying. The health benefits are so enormous that it's well-worth seeing it through.

"I had been a smoker for 29 years and thoroughly enjoyed my bad habit. However, I knew it was unwise, and every now and then I'd decide to give up. Over the years I tried hypnotherapy, patches, gum and willpower, but nothing worked – the desire to smoke was just too strong.

Then I had a bit of a shock. I broke a bone in my wrist at the age of 56 and my doctor told me that it was due to osteoporosis. I decided to stop smoking at once, and discovered that when you really want to, it's not that hard to do it.

I wish it hadn't taken a health scare to make me stop, but at least I got around to it eventually. And strangely enough, I feel fitter and stronger now than I did during that thirty years as a much younger smoker!"

Pamela, aged 59

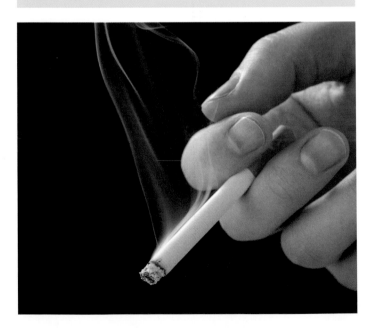

CUT DOWN ON CAFFEINE AND CARBONATED DRINKS

Drinking too much caffeine can be harmful to your bones as it causes your kidneys to get rid of calcium in your urine. Drinking too many carbonated drinks is also harmful because they too prevent calcium from being absorbed by the bones.

Many people drink unhealthy amounts of tea, coffee and caffeinated soft drinks each day. Some caffeine is disguised in other products – coca cola and chocolate contain a certain amount of caffeine, for example. As well as having negative effects on the bones, excess caffeine also causes anxiety, restlessness, palpitations, tremors and shakes. Carbonated drinks usually contain lots of sugar (which damages your teeth and piles on the pounds) and have no other nutritional benefits whatsoever.

It is recommended that you eat healthy, caffeine-free snacks – for example fruit – and limit caffeinated drinks to two per day or choose healthier alternatives such as:

- De-caffeinated drinks
- Fruit juice (but not too much, as this also contains sugar)
- Herbal and fruit teas
- Water! – it offers the body more hydration and is more refreshing and healthy

HABIT REPLACEMENT

Most of us struggle to stop our less healthy habits and we can often experience a feeling of withdrawal that can contribute to the habit taking over the mind. An alternative strategy that may work is to focus on increasing your healthy habits instead. Another suggestion is to replace or swap some of the unhealthier habits (some of the time) with healthier habits:

- Eat a piece of fruit instead of having a cup of coffee.

- Drink a glass of water instead of a carbonated drink.

- Go for a short walk instead of having a cigarette.

- Practise breathing exercises (page 53) instead of having a cigarette.

- Relax or meditate for 5 minutes before or instead of having a glass of wine.

Try to make a list of some of the issues that trigger unhealthy habits such as reaching for a chocolate bar, a drink or a cigarette, and think about some strategies that can be used to overcome them.

It takes around 21 days to break a habit – or to set a new one – so you need a bit of perseverance. The first couple of weeks are going to be the hardest, but things do get easier if you don't try to change everything overnight. Remember, you only need to change one thing at a time!

> Habit is habit, and not to be flung out of the window, but coaxed downstairs a step at a time.
>
> **Mark Twain**

> ## GET A GOOD NIGHT'S SLEEP

If you struggle to sleep well, the following tips may help to break a cycle of poor sleeping:

- Make sure your bed and bedroom are at a comfortable temperature and not too noisy or light.

- If you can't sleep, the main thing is not to lie there getting frustrated but to get up and do something relaxing. Read a book or listen to quiet music. After a while you should feel sleepy and relaxed enough to go back to bed.

- Keep to regular sleeping times – i.e. try to get to bed at the same time every night.

- Have a relaxing bath to help you to unwind before you go to bed. Water provides a comforting sensation for the body and soft lighting is restful for the eyes. Candles can be used as focus for meditation – you can watch the flame 'dance'.

- Make sure your mattress is comfy and supports you well. Change it every 10 years or so.

- Keep a notebook by your bed so that you can write down any thoughts that disrupt your sleeping patterns.

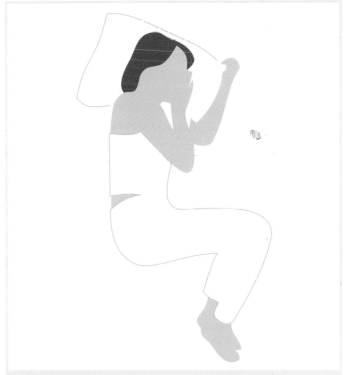

Sleep and rest are part of a healthy lifestyle. A bad night's sleep can leave you tired and make you vulnerable to falls.

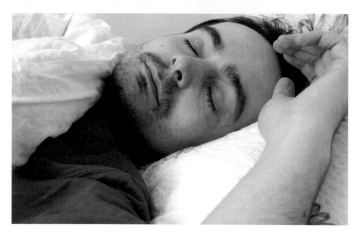

- Keep the bedroom for sleeping, rather than watching television or other activities.

- Try some relaxation or meditation before you go to bed.

- Listen to a relaxation tape or audio book when you go to bed to help you drift off to sleep.

- Allow a couple of hours after exercising before you go to bed.

- Aim to save your sleeping time for bedtime, rather than napping during the day.

- Only drink fluids without stimulants (water, herbal tea) close to bedtime; try to avoid caffeine and alcohol.

- Eat an early evening meal so that you are not eating too close to bedtime.

- If you smoke, allow a couple of hours between your last cigarette and going to bed.

> **BREATHING FOCUS**
Correct breathing enables us to take more oxygen into the lungs. It can also help to keep our spine mobile, so it is useful to practise this regularly, whatever we are doing.

Breathing exercise

- Start by finding an open posture position (seated in a chair or standing) – see page 65
- Focus awareness on the depth, speed and feeling of your breathing
- Close your eyes or focus on a specific spot looking forwards or slightly downwards (make sure your posture doesn't change)
- Take the breath slightly deeper into the lower rib cage (most people take very shallow breaths into the upper chest area only)
- Keep the breath soft, smooth and rhythmical
- Find a natural breathing pace and power (not forcing or straining)
- Let the breath become effortless and allow it to flow freely
- Notice your abdomen rise and fall
- Allow your lower rib cage to expand sideways (you can place your hands around the ribs if it helps)
- Allow a few minutes just to focus on the breathing and stillness

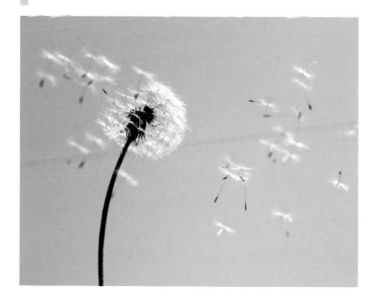

RELAXATION

It is essential to take time out to relax the mind. Relaxation can be a brilliant way to start and end the day – it offers an opportunity for the mind and body to recover fully. It can provide much needed rest and recovery.

Dr Herbert Benson proposed the following method of relaxation to treat patients with high blood pressure. He suggested that individuals sit still and quietly focus on their breathing and, on every outward breath, say out loud the word 'one'. This word can be replaced by other words that you find more natural, such as 'calm' or 'relax' or 'om'. It is possible to use the technique while sitting, standing or lying during everyday activities, for example when queuing at a supermarket, travelling on the train, sitting at an office desk or walking.

- Sit quietly with an open body posture
- Focus on your breathing
- As you breathe out, focus on a desired word
- The word chosen can be spoken out loud or quietly within
- Practise this for about 5–10 minutes, just allowing the body to relax

MEDITATION

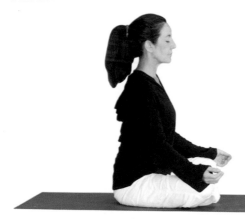

Every day, try to take time to sit quietly for five minutes or so and let unwanted or distracting thoughts pass by. Focus on your breathing and stillness. Any time will do and whenever you can – once the kids are in bed, just before you get up in the morning, or at lunchtime in the corner of a quiet park. Meditation is a great way of relaxing your mind and refreshing yourself.

A treat for your overworked mind

- Sit comfortably, back straight and supported, shoulders relaxed and arms resting on your lap
- Close your eyes
- Focus on breathing deeply and slowly for 10 counts
- Become aware of the activity of the mind and the speed of your thoughts
- Let the thoughts pass through the mind – let them go
- Focus on stillness
- Allow the mind to slow down
- Allow the mind to become quiet and silent
- Let go of other thoughts, acknowledge them, smile and release them
- Keep your focus on stillness
- Keep your focus on your breathing
- Allow the mind to rest
- Allow the mind to be free and peaceful

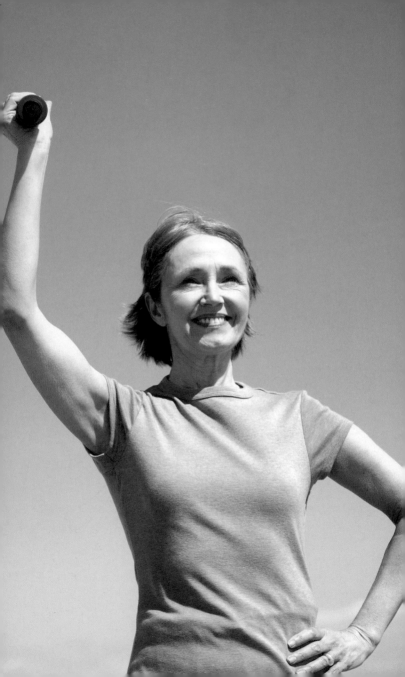

part

3

the exercises

>> Introduction to exercise

This section contains several series of exercises that can be done in your own home. They are designed to help combat the development of osteoporosis. Whatever your level of fitness, some of these will be suitable for you.

There are chair-based exercises for people who want to begin very gently and who need support. If you have kyphosis (rounded upper back), or are anxious about falling, then these are ideal for you. There are also more vigorous exercises for those who are a bit stronger and more confident. You can exercise for any length of time, between 5 and 45 minutes – the emphasis is always on going at your own pace and staying in your comfort zone.

There is plenty of information about exercise and osteoporosis, guidance on posture – whether seated or standing – and tips and suggestions to help you exercise safely and effectively. Please read the section through before you get started. Ideally an exercise programme needs to be balanced. It should include mobility and flexibility exercises, cardiovascular (aerobic-type) activities, and some strength and balance work. The purpose of each type of exercise is outlined below.

MOBILITY AND FLEXIBILITY

- Maintain or improve the flexibility of those muscles that contribute to good posture (e.g. stretching the chest muscles to improve or prevent rounded-back posture).
- Maintain good ranges of movement to keep you flexible throughout the whole body.

CARDIOVASCULAR

- Use weight-bearing activities, such as walking and marching, to increase the strength of your bones.
- Maintain existing fitness and, where possible, make improvements to cardiovascular or heart health.

STRENGTH AND BALANCE

- Focus on weight-bearing exercises for areas more vulnerable to fractures, such as the wrist, hip, spine and collarbone.

Exercise and osteoporosis

Here are some tips to bear in mind if you are exercising with osteoporosis:

- It's important to strengthen the muscles around the common fracture sites (hip, wrist and spine) to help reduce the risk of fractures.

- If weight-bearing exercise is not possible for you, use chair-based exercises.

- Ensure the environment is free of obstacles to reduce any anxiety or fear you may have about falling.

- Be aware of your posture and work on improving it (see page 65).

- Perform correct breathing exercises regularly (page 53), as these help to mobilise your spine and reduce stiffness.

- A combination of strength work for the lower body and balance work will decrease the risk of falls.
- Improve posture and maintain the strength of the vertebral bones. Strength exercises for the midsection, such as the abdominals and back muscles, are vital.
- Strengthening the muscles that help to straighten the back is particularly important, as these muscles act as a splint to protect the spine.

DIFFERENT WAYS TO EXERCISE

There are three main ways to exercise and these are listed below. This book focuses mainly on exercises you can do in the privacy of your own home, at your convenience, but it's worth bearing in mind that there are other options and that these carry their own benefits. Exercise classes can be stimulating and sociable occasions, while outdoor exercise – even if it's just a gentle walk – can lift your mood, even as the daylight stimulates your production of the all-important vitamin D.

1. SUPERVISED SESSIONS

Find out what exercise options are available to you locally in a community hall, leisure centre or health club. There will often be a range of classes – from chair-based exercises, gentle tai chi and Pilates, to more vigorous step and dance sessions. It is best to discuss your needs with an exercise professional first – he or she can advise on the option that is best for you.

You also need to find an activity you really *like* doing; this ensures that you will look forward to the sessions and be much more likely to carry on doing them on a regular basis. Activities such as step, aerobics, ballroom dancing, toning classes and Pilates (which should focus on posture, balance and strengthening your core muscles) will be helpful.

2. GO OUTDOORS

Exercising outdoors offers many positive benefits for our mood and mental health. It also offers an opportunity for us to receive our daily dose of vitamin D. Walking itself is extremely good for you. If you are mobile enough, you could join a group like the ramblers, or find a local walking group. If you're less mobile, a gentle walk to the shops, round the park or up the road and back will still have real benefits.

Spend time outdoors

Being outdoors, especially in sunshine, boosts our vitamin D levels – essential for strong bones – so make sure you regularly go outside, particularly during the summer months. In very hot weather when the sun is shining, in hot countries or at times of day when the sun is stronger, everyone should use a sunscreen to avoid sunburn, especially if you have sensitive or pale skin. This will keep your skin safe and prevent skin damage caused by ultraviolet rays.

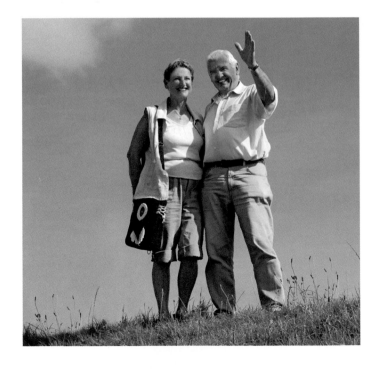

We have a natural connection to the outdoor environment and being outdoors can help us to feel more content and function more effectively. Being in a natural environment can help the brain to recharge, refocus and relax.

As with all exercise though, you should take care only to do what is safe and comfortable for you, so if you have advanced kyphosis (a rounded upper spine) then you will be better remaining indoors and doing the chair-based exercises on page 71. If in doubt you could always take a companion with you on your first outing.

3. HOME EXERCISE

The benefit of exercising at home is that you can fit it in at any time that suits you, either with short sessions throughout the day, or putting aside 30 minutes at a time. The biggest difficulty is getting into a regular pattern.

On the plus side, home exercise is cheap and you don't have to leave the house on a cold, wet day – or you can exercise in the garden when the sun is shining.

A lot of the exercises can be done when you are watching TV or even lying in bed, or you can put on some music you love, which can really get you going.

> We have a weekly chair-based exercise class at the residential home where I live. I have been attending for a year. When I first started, I had to use my hands to help push me out of the chair, but now I can get out of the chair without holding on. My legs are stronger and so is my tummy – my balance has improved too. The overall result is that I feel stronger and more stable than I have for ten years!

Margaret, aged 86

More tips for exercising

- Wear loose comfortable clothing and a supportive pair of trainers.

- If you are exercising outdoors, make sure you wear appropriate clothing and use sunscreen in summer.

- Take a mobile phone if exercising outdoors, and tell someone where you are going.

- If you feel thirsty, sip water throughout but avoid taking long drinks.

- If you have eaten a heavy meal, wait two hours before exercising.

- If you feel hungry, have a light snack like a banana or a piece of toast.

- If anything feels uncomfortable, then stop doing it.

- Move any chairs, tables or bags out of the way.

- Check rugs and carpets to make sure there is nothing you can trip on.

- Breathe naturally at all times – don't hold your breath.

- Always complete the warm-up before you perform other exercises.

- Try to stretch gently afterwards.

- Never force yourself to do anything that causes you pain.

- If you feel dizzy or uncomfortable, stop at once.

- Ask someone to be with you if you are unsure it's safe to exercise alone.

- Music or a friend to exercise with can motivate you.

> > Start safely

Before you start, take some steps to make sure you are exercising safely. First work out which level of exercise is right for you by following the instructions on page 27. Then complete the questionnaire on page 30. If you answered yes to any of the questions, you should check with a GP before starting to exercise.

It's always best to start exercising at a gentle level and gradually work harder as you grow more confident. Remember that even if it's just five minutes a day it's still doing you good.

If you think you are at risk of osteoporosis or have been diagnosed, then the movements listed below, especially if you have kyphosis:

- Bending forwards
- Touching your toes
- Circling your head backwards
- Bouncing when stretching (you should hold stretches and use smooth movements)
- Twisting 180 degrees, which can make you dizzy and put a strain on your hips and back
- High-impact exercises such as jumping and running
- Lying down on your back

> GETTING SAFELY TO THE FLOOR AND UP AGAIN

It is important that we all maintain our ability to get down to and up from the floor – especially if we are at risk of falling. As the saying goes 'use it or lose it', so do practise doing this from time to time. If it seems daunting, think about it as a series of small steps. Work your way through them slowly, taking time to feel comfortable in each position before moving on to the next. Then work your way back up again to a standing position.

If you haven't been down to floor-level recently you might want to have someone else present when you attempt this. Note: don't attempt this for 12 months after a hip fracture or hip replacement.

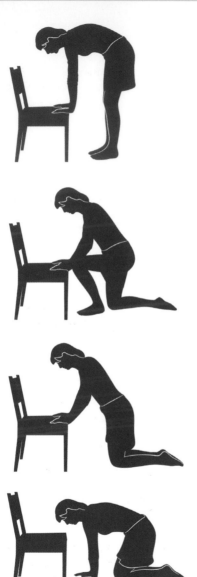

1. Firstly, place both hands on the seat of a chair.

2. Bend one knee so you are half kneeling on the floor. Don't place the knee too close to the chair itself.

3. Lower the other knee to the floor, using your hands for support.

4. Now move your hands to the floor so you are on 'all fours'.

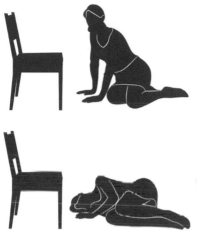

5. Gently lower your hips to the side so they are resting on the floor.

6. And lower the rest of your body to the floor.

>> Posture

Standing and moving with correct posture not only gives the impression of greater confidence but can actually *lead* to increased confidence. It's also much better for your health:

- Good posture helps the body function well.

- Poor posture can cause stress on the muscles, particularly in the lower back.

- It can also lead to shallow and ineffective breathing.

- A slumped posture can affect the inner organs and digestion.

- Bad posture can lead to permanent problems that cause pain or instability.

It is much better to begin your exercises from a position of good posture. It makes the exercise both more effective and safer. For this reason, take some time to practise good posture, both seated and standing. Here is some guidance to help you.

SEATED POSTURE

You could ask someone to check how you are sitting or sit in front of a mirror if you are not sure. It is important to sit correctly to prevent low back pain – sitting correctly also enables us to breathe more fully.

- Sit towards the front of a chair
- Place your feet parallel and hip-width apart, with knees over ankles
- Distribute your weight evenly between your heel bone, big toe and little toe and spread your toes
- Sit upright and lengthen your spine as much as you can
- Lift out of your sitting bones to find a neutral spine position (pubic bone and hip bones in line to ensure no or minimal forward or backward tilt of pelvis)
- Lengthen your torso and neck
- Tighten your abdominals by breathing in your stomach muscles
- Look forwards, keeping your chin parallel to the floor
- Keeping your shoulders relaxed and down, slide your shoulder blades down
- Place your hands by the sides of the chair, palms facing forwards.

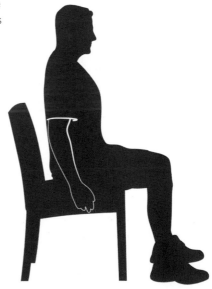

STANDING POSTURE

You can do this in front of a mirror or ask a friend to check how you are standing. Ideally, if you are standing side on to them, they should be able to visualise a straight line running from your ear lobe to the middle of your ankle. Your body should be upright, without leaning back or forwards and without any excessive rounding or hollowing of the spine.

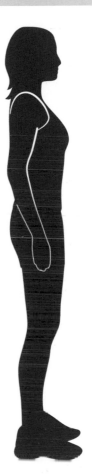

- Stand with your feet parallel and hip-width apart
- Distribute your weight between heel bone, big toe and little toe
- Spread your toes, aligning second toe with knee and hip
- Find a neutral spine position, see below
- Lengthen your torso and neck
- Tighten your tummy muscles by imagining you're zipping up a tight pair of trousers
- Look forwards, keeping your chin parallel to the floor
- Keeping your shoulders relaxed and down, slide your shoulder blades down your back
- Keep your hands by the sides of your body, palms facing forwards.

Finding the natural position for your spine

Finding what we call the neutral spine position is very easy. Simply tilt your pelvis gently forwards to curve your back and then gently backwards to hollow your back. Find the middle between these two extremes – this gives you the natural curves in your back.

>> **Are you ready?**

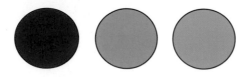

All the exercises that follow are colour-coded – green, amber, red – according to the risk classification you should have worked out in Part 2. Look at the reminder of the classifications opposite.

> Don't forget to look through the questions on pages 29 and 38. Make sure you are fit to get physical.

Chair-based exercises are recommended for frailer adults and those diagnosed with osteoporosis. These are a good starting point for anyone in the amber or red categories. Non-chair-based exercises are applicable to anyone in the green category, and also to those people in the amber category who have completed the chair-based exercises for a few weeks and feel strong enough to move up.

Remember that you should always start slowly, and you should always begin by warming up gently. A warm-down involving some simple stretches is also a good idea.

Even if you think you could do something harder, why not begin with a few simple chair-based exercises and do them for five or ten minutes a few times a week. You can gradually mix in other exercises and create a longer routine that is comfortable for you.

Any exercise is beneficial. If you only manage five minutes a few times a week that is a still good progress. What you are aiming for is regular sessions five days a week, but not everyone can manage this.

Reminder of traffic-light system for risk classification	
No clinical diagnosis	Most of the exercises will be appropriate for you – follow the exercises with the green lights.
	You will need to take account of your current fitness and activity levels and exercise experience – start gradually and build up steadily.
	Some higher-impact work (jumps) can be included during the cardiovascular exercises.
Clinically diagnosed	You may need more care and attention with your chosen activities – follow the exercises with the amber lights but work at an easier level (fewer repetitions and lower intensity).
	Keep any cardiovascular exercises low impact – without a hop.
	Take care with some exercise positions (lying on the back or front) and with weight-bearing joints (wrist).
Frailer groups	Take care! You probably have a lower tolerance of exercise and activity.
	It is likely that you have a fear of falling or have experienced a minor fall.
	Perform exercises that make you feel safe and supported.
	Ideally you should attend a supervised exercise session.
	The chair-based exercise section is most appropriate for you – follow the exercises with the red lights.
	You can practise correct posture and breathing.

Note: All the routines that follow can take more or less time, depending on how many repetitions of each exercise you select and how many cycles of the exercise sequence you choose to perform. Listen to your body, start gently, go for little and often at first, and gradually work your way up. If you find that an exercise causes you pain, stop at once.

Still feeling a bit reluctant? Here's a reminder of the positive benefits of exercise:

- I will have more energy
- My bones will get stronger
- I will feel more cheerful
- My posture will improve
- I will sleep better at night
- I am doing something constructive
- I'm devoting some time to myself
- My breathing will improve

I was running down the stairs to answer the doorbell when I slipped and broke both my ankles. I was only 42 and this was the first sign that I had osteoporosis. I hated being immobile and had to perform some exercises in bed, to keep my muscles strong.

I knew that, if I didn't start building my strength, I could potentially be immobile by the time I was 50, so I started practising a few exercises every day to improve my strength and balance.

I had to hold a wall because my balance was awful at first, and I was terrified about breaking another bone or injuring my weak ankles. But gradually I grew stronger, and now I feel so much steadier on my legs. I know I've improved my chances of remaining independent for a while longer!

Theresa, aged 49

Equipment

It is preferable to use a chair without arms for the seated exercises so that you can move freely.

Instead of dumbbells you could use plastic water bottles – start with an empty bottle and add water to it to increase the weight you lift. Alternatively, holding small tins of baked beans or other canned food can add resistance for arm exercises like biceps curls and triceps extensions.

>> Chair-based exercises

In this section you will find three types of exercise: the warm-up, stretching, and strength and balance. You can do these exercises anytime, anywhere. They offer the support of a chair and, provided you start gently and stop if you are in any discomfort, they should be suitable for all three risk categories.

Choose one exercise or perform them all. The key thing is to start steadily and gradually build up. Always begin with the warm-up exercises, which are very gentle. Do these for between five and ten minutes. When you are comfortable with these exercises you can progress to stretches, then move on to strength and balance. If an exercise feels uncomfortable or if you do not like it, leave it out.

Chair-based warm-up

Suitable for:

These nine exercises are great to get you moving gently. Once you are comfortable doing them, move on to the chair-based stretching exercises. This series of seated exercises should take between five and ten minutes, but go at your own pace.

1. SEATED SHOULDER LIFTS

1️⃣ Sit with your feet hip width apart
2️⃣ Sit upright and tighten the tummy
3️⃣ Lift your shoulders towards your ears
4️⃣ Lower your shoulders and feel your shoulder
   blades slide back down
5️⃣ Repeat 8–12 times

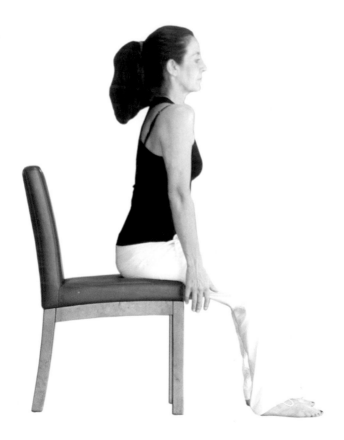

2. SEATED SHOULDER ROLLS

1 Sit with your feet hip width apart
2 Sit upright and tighten the tummy
3 Roll your shoulders forwards, upwards and then backwards and down
4 When lowering, feel your shoulder blades slide towards the buttocks
5 Repeat 8–12 times

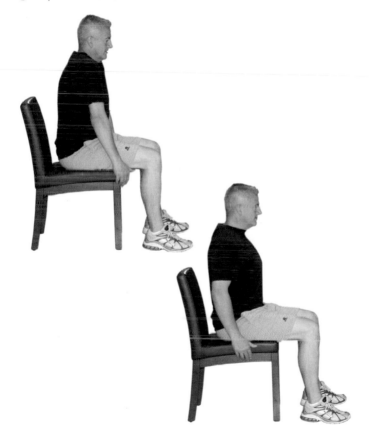

3. SEATED ARM SWINGS

❶ Sit on the front third of the chair with your feet hip width apart
❷ Let your arms hang down by your sides
❸ Sit tall with a straight back and pull in your tummy
❹ Swing one arm forwards to approximately shoulder height
❺ Swing it back behind you as far as is comfortable
❻ Return it to the start position by your side
❼ Do the same with the other arm
❽ Repeat 8–20 times on alternate arms

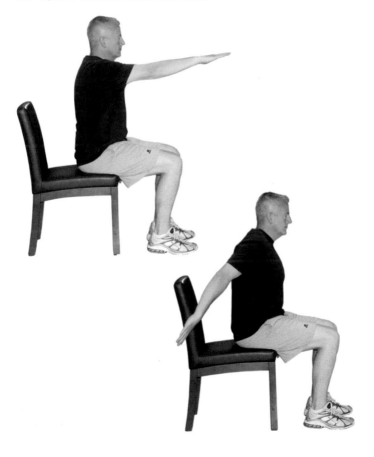

4. SEATED HEEL–TOE

1 Sit on the front third of the chair

2 Dig the heel of the foot towards the floor with the toes lifting upwards

3 Then point the toe towards the floor, and lift the heel away from the floor

4 Aim for the heel and toe to land in the same place to ensure the full range of motion in the ankle is achieved

5 Repeat on the other leg

6 Repeat 8–12 times on each foot

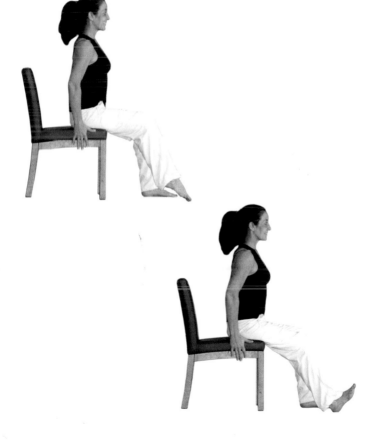

5. SEATED SIDE BENDS

1. Sit with your feet hip width apart and your body upright
2. Pull in your tummy and lift the chest
3. Bend to the side without leaning forwards or back – you may not be able to go very far
4. Return to the central position
5. Remember to lift and bend in a controlled manner, and only as far over as is comfortable
6. Repeat 8–12 times

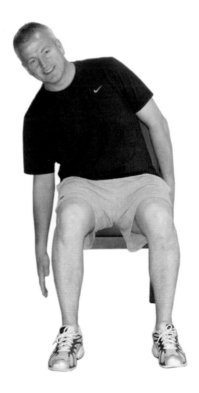

6. SEATED ARM OPENING

❶ Sit with your feet hip width apart
❷ Maintain an upright posture and tuck in your tummy
❸ Bring both arms to cross in front of you at chest level, or lower if you prefer
❹ Smoothly and gently open both arms out to the sides and slightly back
❺ Return your arms to the front and repeat
❻ Remember to keep your tummy tucked in and your back straight throughout
❼ Perform 8–12 repetitions

Note: you can do this exercise one arm at a time if you prefer.

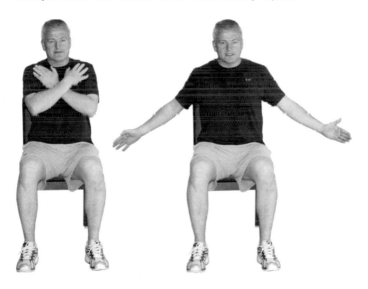

7. SEATED SIDE TWISTS

1 Sit with your feet hip-width apart
2 Maintain an upright posture, tuck in your tummy and rest your arms comfortably
3 Twist around to one side
4 Turn back to centre
5 Twist around to the other side
6 Remember to keep your chest lifted and your shoulders relaxed
7 Repeat 8–12 times

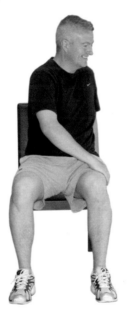

Note: if you are performing this exercise standing, keep your hips facing forward throughout the exercise – you twist from the waist, not the hips.

8. SEATED MARCHING

1 Sit on the front third of the chair with your feet hip-width apart
2 Sit tall with a straight back and pull in your tummy
3 Peel your foot off the floor and lift your leg so your foot is a few inches off the floor
4 Lightly put your foot back down again
5 Do the same on the other leg
6 Remember to breath naturally throughout
7 Repeat on alternate legs 8–20 times

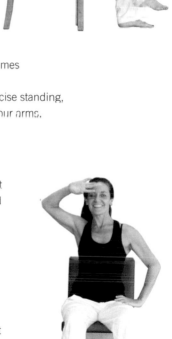

Note: if you are performing this exercise standing, feel free to move about and swing your arms.

9. SEATED ARM CIRCLES

1 Sit with your feet hip-width apart
2 Maintain an upright posture and tuck in your tummy
3 Gentle circle your right arm in front of you, over the head and behind
4 Repeat on the left side
5 Remember to start with a small circle – almost like brushing the hair – and keep your elbow bent
6 Repeat 8–12 times

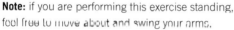

Chair-based stretches

Suitable for:

If you have completed your warm-up, you can now move on to stretches. It is important that you feel warm before stretching, as this prevents injury. These four stretches should take between five and ten minutes, but as always you should go at your own pace.

1. SEATED BACK OF THIGH STRETCH

1 Sit upright with your feet hip-width apart, knees bent and tummy pulled in

2 Straighten one leg out to the front, keeping in straight but not locked

3 Place your hands on the chair for support

4 Bend forwards from the hip until a mild tension is felt at the back of your thigh

5 Hold the stretch for 8–12 seconds, trying to keep your spine long and your chest lifted

6 Return to your starting position and repeat on the other side

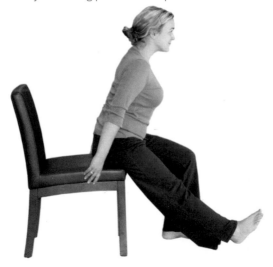

2. SEATED CHEST STRETCH

1. Sit upright with your feet hip-width apart and pull in your tummy
2. Hold the back of the chair with both hands – or you can place them on your buttocks or clasp them behind your back
3. Lean forwards slightly until a mild tension is felt at the front of the chest
4. Keep your elbows slightly bent
5. Squeeze your shoulder blades together and lift your chest to increase the stretch
6. Hold the stretch for 8–12 seconds

3. SEATED CALF STRETCH

1. Sit on the front third of your chair
2. Sit upright with your feet hip-width apart, knees bent and tummy pulled in
3. Straighten one leg out to the front, keeping the knee unlocked
4. Flex the foot so your toes point upwards
5. Hold the stretch for 8–12 seconds
6. Repeat on the other leg

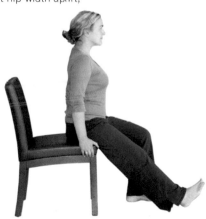

4. SEATED ARM LIFT AND BEND

1 Sit upright with your feet hip-width apart
2 Place one arm on the side of the chair to support your body weight
3 Lift your other arm up
4 Bend over slightly towards the side with the supporting arm
5 Stretch only to a point where a mild tension is felt at the side of the trunk
6 Keep a space between your shoulders and your ears and lengthen your neck
7 Remember to lengthen your neck and don't lean forwards or back
8 It helps to lift your rib cage upwards and create a gap between your pelvis and your ribs before bending to the side
9 Hold the stretch for 8–12 seconds
10 Repeat on the other side

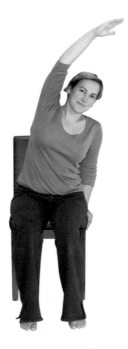

Chair-based strength and balance

Suitable for:

This is the last series of exercises in the chair-based exercise set. You should not undertake any of these exercises unless you have completed the warm-up and ideally the stretches. Make sure you feel warm before you begin. These exercises should take between 10 and 15 minutes but remember that the number of repetitions here is just a guide – it's important to start gently and build up step by step. Do what you feel comfortable with and go at your own pace.

1. SEATED LEG KICKS

1 Sit upright with your feet hip-width apart and pull in your tummy

2 Try to lengthen one leg in front of you until it straightens, lifting your foot from the floor

3 Bend the knee and place the foot back on the floor and repeat with your other leg

4 Repeat 4–12 times on each leg

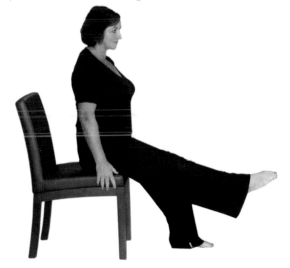

2. SEATED CHEST PRESS

① Sit upright with your feet hip-width apart and pull in your tummy
② Press both arms forward at chest level, arms straight and the heel of your hand outwards
③ Bring your elbows back into your waist
④ Repeat 8–12 times

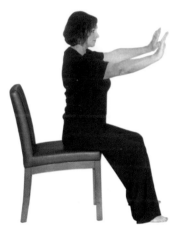

3. SEATED LIFT AND RAISE

① Sit on the front third of the chair with a good upright posture
② Rest your hands lightly on top of your thighs
③ Keep the chest lifted and lengthen the back
④ Engage your abdominals by pulling in your tummy muscles
⑤ Hold your tummy in for a count of four
⑥ Release back to the starting position
⑦ Repeat 4–12 times

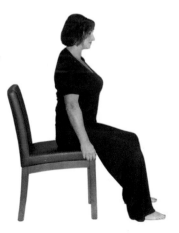

4. SEATED CHIN TUCKS AND NECK TILTS

1. Sit on the front third of the chair with a good upright posture
2. Tuck your chin in to make as many double chins as you can
3. Hold for a count of five and then release
4. Perform 8–12 repetitions
5. Then turn your head as far as you can to the right, then to the left
6. Then tilt your head over so your right ear is aiming for your right shoulder

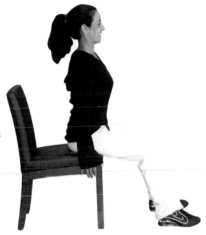

7. Finally tilt your head over so your left ear aims for your left shoulder
8. Bring your head back to the centre and rest

5. SEATED MIDDLE BACK

1. Sit tall so your bottom almost touches the back of the chair
2. Rest your hands on your thighs
3. Lift your chest and tighten your abdominal muscles
4. Lean slightly back until your shoulder blades touch the back of the chair
5. Return to the starting position
6. Remember to breathe naturally and keep your back straight and your chin tucked in
7. Repeat 4–12 times

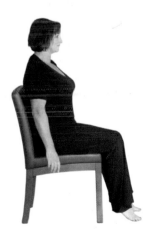

6. SEATED WRING AND PULL

❶ Sit tall on the front third of the chair with a good upright posture
❷ Hold a rolled-up towel in your hands, with one hand above the other
❸ Rotate your two hands in opposite directions as though wringing the towel
❹ Pull your hands apart slightly before returning them to the starting position
❺ Repeat 8 times

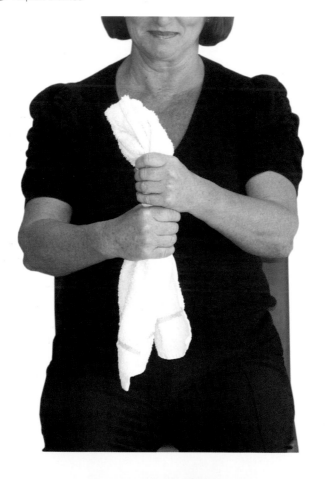

7. SIT TO STAND

Purpose: This is a useful exercise that should be performed on its own, not necessarily as part of an exercise regime, on a regular basis. Standing from a sitting position often grows harder with age, so it is strongly recommended that older readers practise this essential skill.

1. Sit on the front third of the chair with a good upright posture
2. Rest your hands lightly on the sides of the chair
3. It may help to place one foot slightly in front of the other
4. Either pushing with your arms or just using your legs, lift up your whole body to a standing position
5. Lower yourself back to the seat with control
6. Repeat, building up to 8–10 times if you can

Note: this is a hard exercise because you are using all your body weight, so start gently and build up gradually. Make sure someone supervises you if you have mobility problems and normally experience difficulty moving from sitting to standing.

> > Standing exercises

In this section you will find four types of exercise: the warm-up, stretching, cardiovascular exercises, and strength and balance. These are for people who are more mobile and not at risk of falling, so those in the amber and green categories.

You should begin with the warm-up. Next combine the warm-up with some simple stretches. As you grow stronger and fitter, you can add cardio or strength and balance exercises to your routine – or both.

You may find that you are restricted to just a few simple exercises, or you may be able to do them all. You may manage five minutes, or half an hour. As ever, work at your own pace and build up. If anything is uncomfortable you should stop doing it.

Standing warm-up

Suitable for:

Even if you are in the amber or green categories you need to start with a five- to ten-minute warm up before moving on to other exercises. It is important that you start these from a good standing position where your posture is upright and your pelvis in a neutral position (see page 67 for details). Your feet should be just over shoulder-width apart. Always try to maintain the length of the spine and neck in your exercises. Keep your feet firmly on the ground, and if concerned about your balance, hold on to the back of a chair or stay close to a wall for support. Breathe naturally while you exercise and don't hold your breath. If you like, you can combine seated and standing warm-up exercises, doing some of each.

1. SHOULDER ROLLS

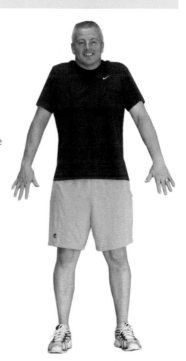

❶ Gently roll your shoulders forwards, then up and backwards and finally downwards

❷ As you lower your shoulders, feel your shoulder blades slide down towards your buttocks

❸ Perform 8–12 repetitions

2. SIDE BENDS

❶ Bend directly to the side in a controlled manner and return to the central position

❷ Bend directly to the other side in a controlled manner and return to the central position

❸ Visualise your body as being placed between two panes of glass and bend only as far over as is comfortable

❹ Keep your hips facing forwards and the movement controlled

❺ Keep your body lifted between the hips and the ribs

❻ Perform 8–16 repetitions on each side (alternating)

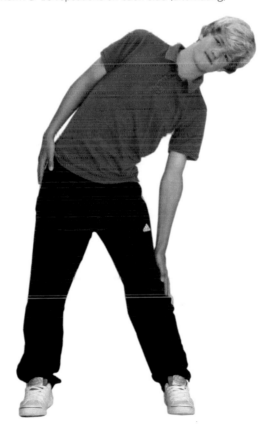

3. SIDE TWISTS

1. Start with your feet shoulder width and a half apart
2. Hold out your arms at shoulder level, with your elbows slightly bent or place your hands on hips
3. Twist your arms around to one side, back to the centre and then twist to the other side
4. Twist only as far around as is comfortable
5. Keep your hips and knees facing forwards
6. Perform 8–16 repetitions on each side (alternating)

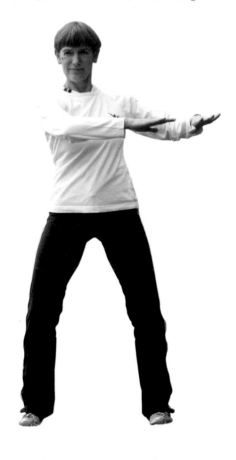

4. HEEL AND TOE

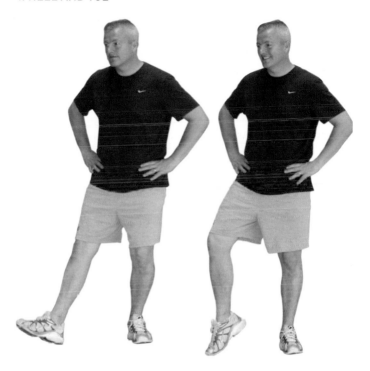

1. Start with your feet shoulder width and a half apart and take your weight onto one leg
2. Dig the heel of your free foot towards the floor and then point the toe towards the floor
3. Keep your weight-bearing leg soft, your hips facing forwards and the movement controlled
4. Aim for the heel and toe to land in the same place
5. Repeat on the other leg
6. Perform 8–16 repetitions on each side (alternating)

5. KNEE LIFTS

1. Start with your feet shoulder width and a half apart
2. Start raising alternate knees in front of your body
3. Take a comfortable stride of the legs
4. Keep your hips facing forwards
5. Lift your leg only to a height where an upright spine alignment can be maintained
6. Keep your chest lifted and do not allow your body to bend forwards as your leg lifts
7. Perform for 1–2 minutes

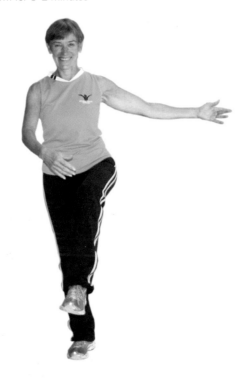

6. WALKING OR MARCHING

1 Start with your feet shoulder width and a half apart
2 Maintain an upright posture and engage your abdominals
3 Start marching or walking on the spot
4 Land your feet lightly
5 Keep your knees unlocked
6 You can play music and march/walk for longer periods
7 You can also travel this movement forwards and backwards or around the room
8 Perform for 2–4 minutes

Note: Marching and walking can be used as a warm-up in their own right. They will raise your heart rate and warm your muscles. These movements can also be used between exercises, or between repetitions of exercises, as you build up strength and stamina.

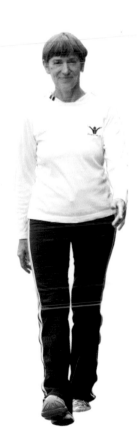

7. SQUATS WITH ARM CIRCLES

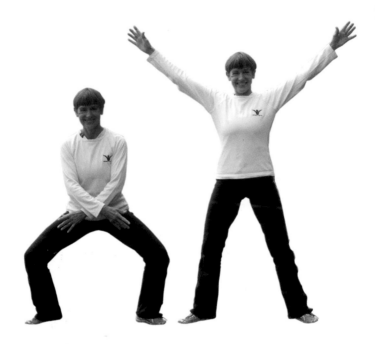

1 Start with your feet two hip-widths apart, so that when you bend your knees they stay in line with your toes
2 Bend your knees to a 90-degree angle
3 Straighten your legs without locking your knees
4 Add a circling movement of your arms in front of your body to raise the intensity
5 Start with 30 seconds and then march for 30 seconds
6 Gradually build up the time to match your level of comfort

Standing stretches

Suitable for:

Complete the warm-up before tackling these five stretches so that your muscles are nice and warm. This is to avoid any injuries while stretching. As ever, only do what is comfortable and try to breathe steadily throughout. You should also return to these stretches for the warm down, after you have completed the cardio and/or strength and balance exercises. Go at your own pace, and stretch gently at first.

1. HAMSTRINGS STRETCH

1. Start with your feet shoulder width apart
2. Maintain an upright posture and pull in your tummy
3. Step forwards – a shoulder-width stride
4. Bend the back knee and rest your hands lightly on the thigh of the bent leg
5. Your other leg should be extended in front of you but don't lock the knee
6. Bend forwards from the hips, supporting your weight with the hand on your bent leg, until a mild tension is felt at the back of your straight leg
7. Hold the stretch for 10–12 seconds
8. Remember to keep your weight-bearing knee slightly bent and facing forwards, and keep your spine long and your chest lifted
9. Repeat on the other leg

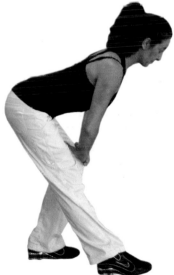

2. QUADRICEPS STRETCH

1 Maintain an upright posture and pull in your tummy
2 Balance on one leg, using a wall or chair for support – do not lock this knee
3 Raise the heel of the opposite leg towards your buttocks
4 Use your hand to hold the leg in place, making sure that it's towards the centre of your body and not out to the side
5 Hold the stretch for 10–12 seconds
6 Remember to keep your hips facing forwards and your body lifted
7 Repeat on the other leg

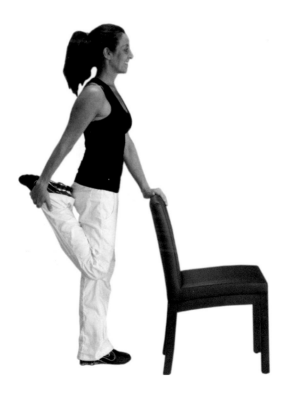

3. CALF STRETCH

① Start with your feet just over shoulder width apart
② Maintain an upright posture and pull in your tummy
③ Step your right leg backwards
④ Make sure the heel of your back foot is on the floor
⑤ Your front knee should bend forwards gently until you feel tension in your back calf
⑥ Use a wall for support if you need to
⑦ Hold the stretch for 10–12 seconds
⑧ Repeat on the other leg

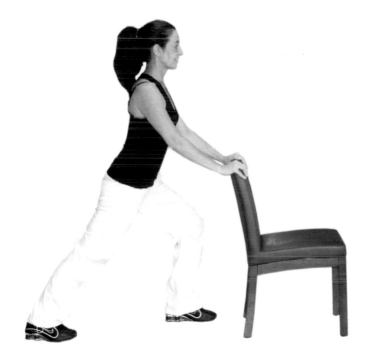

4. TRICEPS STRETCH

1. Start with your feet just over shoulder width apart and your knees slightly bent
2. Maintain an upright posture and pull in your tummy
3. Lift one arm up, bend it and place the hand in the centre of your back
4. Use your other arm to ease the arm further down until you feel a mild tension at the back of your upper arm
5. Hold the stretch for 10–12 seconds
6. Remember to keep your hips facing forwards, and avoid hollowing your lower back by tucking your buttocks under and pulling your tummy in
7. Repeat on the other arm

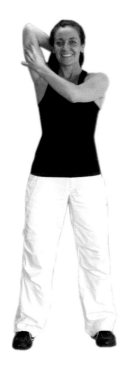

5. CHEST STRETCH

1 Start with your feet just over shoulder width apart, knees unlocked

2 Maintain an upright posture and pull in your tummy

3 Take your hands backwards until a mild tension is felt at the front of your chest, placing them at the top of your buttocks or clasped together behind you, whichever is most comfortable

4 Keep your elbows slightly bent

5 Slide your shoulder blades down towards your buttocks and slightly back

6 Lift your chest to increase the stretch

7 Hold the stretch for 10–12 seconds

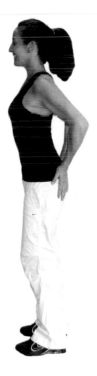

Cardiovascular workout

Suitable for:

These five cardiovascular exercises are weight bearing, which is good for building strong bones and a great way to combat the development of osteoporosis. They involve more movement than the other exercises, so it's important to make sure you have clear space around you. Check the floor area for electrical wires and corners of rugs that might trip you up. You should start gently, work a little harder in the middle of the routine and then ease off. Use marching or jogging on the spot to keep you warm and mobilised between exercises, and to give you a rest between repetitions of the same exercise.

Essential tips for cardio exercises:

- Always start gently and skip any exercises that seem too vigorous
- Make sure you warm up and stretch before a cardiovascular workout
- Stretch again afterwards while you're still nice and warm
- Make sure you rehydrate afterwards
- Don't perform these exercises on a very hard surface like concrete
- Take extra care if you have a joint or muscle problem
- You can march on the spot before and between exercises to keep you warm
- Remember the repetitions are a guide – do what is comfortable and build up

1. SIDE STEPS AND CLAPS

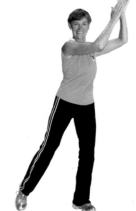

❶ Stand tall with your chest proud
❷ Take a large step to the side and your arms out to the side
❸ Bring your feet together and clap
❹ Repeat the movement to return to the starting position
❺ Start with 30 seconds and then march for 30 seconds

2. LEG CURLS

1 Start with your feet just over shoulder width apart

2 Maintain an upright posture and pull in your tummy

3 Step out to one side and transfer your weight onto that leg

4 Kick your other leg up behind you towards your buttocks

5 Step to the other side as you lower the leg and repeat

6 Remember to keep the movement controlled and smooth

7 Repeat 8 20 times

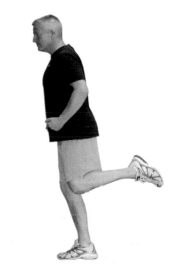

3. KNEE LIFTS AND TWIST

1 Start with your feet just over shoulder width apart

2 Maintain an upright posture and pull in your tummy

3 Start raising alternate knees in front of your body

4 Simultaneously bring a hand towards its opposite raised knee

5 Lift your leg only to a height where you can stay upright

6 Keep your chest lifted and do not allow your body to bend forwards as your leg lifts

7 Repeat 8–12 times

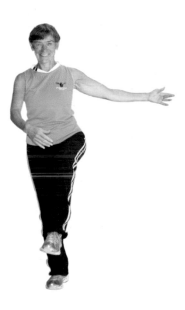

4. SIDE SQUATS

1. Maintain an upright posture and engage your abdominals
2. Lace your hands loosely in front of you or hold them out to the sides
3. Lunge one leg to the side and back together
4. Repeat on the opposite side
5. Remember to keep your knee joints unlocked and in line with your feet, and your hips facing forwards
6. Start with 30 seconds and then go march or jog for 30 seconds, then build up

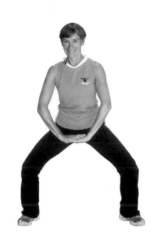

5. LEG KICKS

1. Maintain an upright posture and engage your abdominals
2. Kick alternate legs out in front of your body
3. You can add a small hop as you do so if it feels comfortable
4. Keep your hopping knee joint unlocked and make sure your heel goes down
5. Take care not to lock the knee of your kicking leg
6. Start with 30 seconds of leg kicks and then march for 30 seconds
7. Repeat and gradually build up the time as you grow stronger

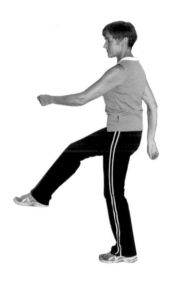

Standing strength and balance

Suitable for:

It is essential to perform five minutes of warm-up exercises before doing this routine. Remember not to hold your breath. If you breathe out on the effort – the lifting phase of the movement – and breathe in on the lowering phase, this will help you. When you have finished the following six exercises, stretch all the muscles while you are nice and warm. If you are worried about your balance hold onto the back of a chair.

1. CALF RAISE

1 Stand behind a sturdy chair and rest your hands on the back of it

2 Place your feet hip width apart

3 Raise onto your toes and lower to the starting point

4 Keep an upright posture throughout

5 Repeat 8–12 times

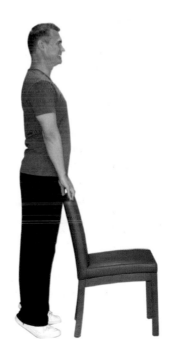

2. KNEE LIFT

1 Stand side on to the chair with your hand resting on it
2 Lengthen your spine and pull in your tummy
3 Lift the knee nearest to the chair
4 See if you can your thigh parallel to the floor
5 Lower the leg
6 Repeat 8–12 times then turn around and exercise the other leg

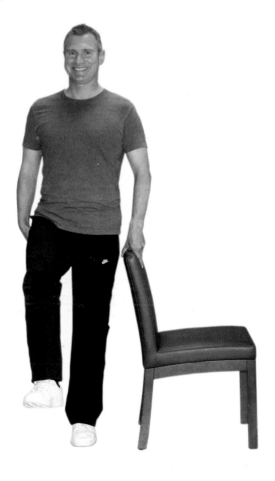

3. SIDE LEG RAISE

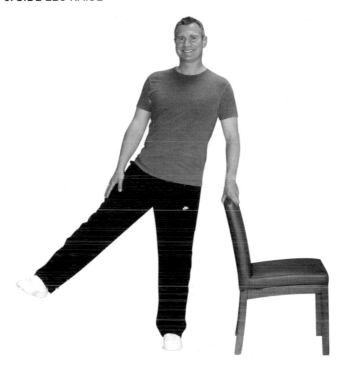

① Stand side on to the chair with your inside hand resting on it
② Lengthen your spine and suck in your abdominals
③ Raise one leg to the side, keeping your hips facing forwards
④ Lower your leg under control
⑤ Perform 8–12 repetitions then repeat on the other leg

4. RHOMBOID SQUEEZE

1 Raise your arms to chest height
2 Take your elbows back, bending them to 90 degrees
3 Stop when you feel a squeeze inbetween your shoulder blades
4 Release slightly
5 Repeat 8–12 times

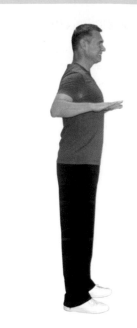

5. UPRIGHT ROW WITH WEIGHTS

1 Use dumbbells or improvised weights like a can of baked beans
2 Stand with your feet hip width apart and your knees slightly bent
3 Lift up the weights to chest level, keeping them close to your body
4 Try to keep elbows raised above your wrists
5 Lower them down under control
6 Start with 8 repetitions and gradually build up to 16–24

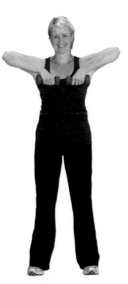

6. BICEPS CURL

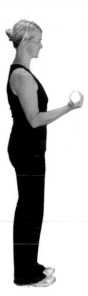

1 Use dumbbells or improvised weights like a can of baked beans

2 Stand with your feet hip width apart

3 Fix your elbows in to the sides of your body

4 Raise the dumbbells in an arc-like motion towards your chest

5 Lower them under control without locking your elbows

6 Keep your wrists fixed and straight

7 Your lower arms should be the only body parts moving

8 Perform one arm at a time if you prefer

9 Start with 8–12 repetitions and gradually build up to 16–24

Thank you for reading

We hope you feel inspired by this book to exercise a little more, and have realised how simple it can be. Whether you give yourself ten minutes of chair-based exercises or feel inspired to put on some music and work your way through a half-hour energetic cardio routine, you will start to feel the benefits almost at once.

But exercise at home isn't for everyone. Some people want to get out of the house into the fresh air, or prefer company. You can do some of these exercises as you walk around the park – just make sure you feel nicely warm beforehand. But don't forget that there are other options, like joining a club or a group, walking with a neighbour, taking an aqua aerobics class (see page 109) or simply helping a friend with the gardening. Everything you do with bring a real glow of satisfaction, and it will really help you help yourself to health. And now go and enjoy yourself!

appendices

> > Appendix 1: In the swim

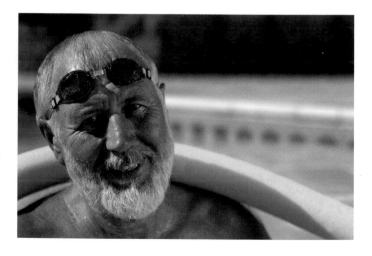

We haven't included swimming in the main part of this book because swimming is not a weight-bearing exercise. However it has a lot of positive health benefits and can be a valuable part of an exercise regime. It can also be extremely gentle since you are supported by the water, and so can be great for people who are recovering from muscle trauma or breaks. Moving around slowly gently exercises your muscles and relaxes you at the same time!

> Care must be taken when walking around a swimming pool, to make sure you don't slip.

Water is a naturally relaxing environment – a hot bath or jacuzzi can have a marvellous effect on relaxing the mind and the muscles. Exercising in water can provide similar relaxing and therapeutic effects. The buoyancy of the water will automatically reduce some of the physical stress on the body. Our body will float and this automatically allows the muscles to relax. The support of the water will reduce any compression of our joints and enable them to move more freely and with greater ease.

The pressure of the water against our body will provide a massaging effect and will promote the circulation of blood and get rid of any unused energy. This will potentially decrease both physical and mental tension, promoting relaxation of the muscles and mind.

If you like swimming, you can start building your swimming routine by starting off with a few widths or lengths and taking short breaks at the end of each one. When you feel ready, you can start taking shorter rests and swimming continuously for longer. Some pools have 'swim fit' cards, which enable you to plan a structured swimming routine to suit your fitness level. You will need to ask one of the pool attendants at your local pool or you can contact one of the swimming organisations, like the amateur swimming association, to get more information on their swim fit programmes.

> > Appendix 2: Write it down!

Here is a log to help you monitor your goals. If you use different colours to represent your changes, you will see the progress you are making. You can use this log to record your progress with any change, whether an exercise regime, a target to increase your activity levels or changes to your diet.

- Start by writing down your current situation as in the example below
- Write down one small change you would like to make on one day
- Make that change and monitor your progress
- When you feel ready, progressively add in more changes on more days

Day / Date	6am–8am	8am–10am	10am–12noon	12noon–2pm	2pm–4pm	4pm–6pm	6pm–8pm	8pm–10pm
Example	Walk to station	Desk exercises		Go for a walk in lunch hour		Walk home from station	Pilates class or swimming	
Monday								
Tuesday								
Wednesday								
Thursday								
Friday								
Saturday								
Sunday								

find out more

OSTEOPOROSIS

National Osteoporosis Society
www.nos.org.uk

Osteoporosis information
www.medinfo.co.uk

Osteoporosis information
www.patient.co.uk

EXERCISE

Exercise for falls prevention
www.laterlifetraining.co.uk

Ramblers
www.getwalking.org

LIFESTYLE

Alcohol Concern
www.alcoholconcern.org.uk

Change4life
www.change4life.com

Food Standards Agency
www.eatwell.gov.uk/healthydiet/eatwellplate

Help the Aged – Preventing Falls Programme
www.helptheaged.org.uk/slipstrips

Smoking cessation
www.quitsmoking.com

bibliography

Benson, H (1975). *The Relaxation Response*. New York. Avon books.

BHF National Centre for Physical Activity and Health (2003). *Active for Later Life*. London. British Heart Foundation.

Bird, W (2007). 'Natural Thinking: A Report for the Royal Society for the Protection of Birds Investigating the Links Between the Natural Environment, Biodiversity and Mental Health'. Available from www.rspb.org.uk.

Bloomfield, S & Smith, S (2003). 'Chapter 34: Osteoporosis'. In Durstine, L J & Moore, G, 2nd Edition, *ACSM's Exercise Management for Persons with Chronic Diseases and Disabilities*. Champaign, USA. Human Kinetics.

British Nutrition Foundation (2005). 'Balance of Good Health'. Available from: www.nutrition.org.uk.

Department of Health (2001). 'Exercise Referral Systems: A National Quality Assurance Framework'. London. Department of Health.

Department of Health (2004). 'At Least Five a Week: Evidence on the Impact of Physical Activity and Its Relationship to Health. A report from the Chief Medical Officer'. London. Department of Health.

Lawrence, D & Barnett, L (2006). *GP Referral Schemes*. London. A&C Black.

National Osteoporosis Society (2006). UK. Available from: www.nos.org.uk.

National Osteoporosis Society (2008). 'All About Osteoporosis'. UK. Available from: www.nos.org.uk.

National Osteoporosis Society (2010). 'Drug Treatment'. UK. Available from: www.nos.org.uk.

PRODIGY (2005). 'Osteoporosis'. UK. Available from: www.prodigy.nhs.uk.